Management of Benign Breast Disease

Editor

MELISSA L. KAPTANIAN

SURGICAL CLINICS
OF NORTH AMERICA

www.surgical.theclinics.com

Consulting Editor
RONALD F. MARTIN

December 2022 • Volume 102 • Number 6

ELSEVIER

1600 John F. Kennedy Boulevard • Suite 1800 • Philadelphia, Pennsylvania, 19103-2899

http://www.surgical.theclinics.com

SURGICAL CLINICS OF NORTH AMERICA Volume 102, Number 6
December 2022 ISSN 0039–6109, ISBN-13: 978-0-323-98733-2

Editor: John Vassallo, j.vassallo@elsevier.com
Developmental Editor: Arlene Campos

Surgical Clinics of North America (ISSN 0039–6109) is published bimonthly by Elsevier Inc., 360 Park Avenue South, New York, NY 10010-1710. Months of publication are February, April, June, August, October, and December. Business and Editorial Offices: 1600 John F. Kennedy Blvd., Suite 1800, Philadelphia, PA 19103-2899. Periodicals postage paid at New York, NY and additional mailing offices. Subscription prices are $456.00 per year for US individuals, $1240.00 per year for US institutions, $100.00 per year for US & Canadian students and residents, $547.00 per year for Canadian individuals, $1283.00 per year for Canadian institutions, $552.00 for international individuals, $1283.00 per year for international institutions and $250.00 per year for foreign students/residents. To receive student/resident rate, orders must be accompanied by name of affiliated institution, date of term, and the *signature* of program/residency coordinator on institution letterhead. Orders will be billed at individual rate until proof of status is received. Foreign air speed delivery is included in all *Clinics* subscription prices. All prices are subject to change without notice. POSTMASTER: Send address changes to *Surgical Clinics*, Elsevier Health Sciences Division, Subscription Customer Service, 3251 Riverport Lane, Maryland Heights, MO 63043. **Customer Service (orders, claims, online, change of address): Telephone: 1-800-654-2452 (U.S. and Canada); 314-447-8871 (outside U.S. and Canada). Fax: 314-447-8029. E-mail: journalscustomerservice-usa@elsevier.com (for print support); journalsonlinesupport-usa@elsevier.com (for online support).**

Reprints. For copies of 100 or more, of articles in this publication, please contact the Commercial Reprints Department, Elsevier Inc., 360 Park Avenue South, New York, New York 10010-1710. Tel. 212-633-3874, Fax: 212-633-3820, E-mail: reprints@elsevier.com.

Surgical Clinics of North America is also published in Spanish by McGraw-Hill Interamericana Editores S.A., P.O. Box 5-237 06500 Mexico D.F. Mexico; and in Portuguese by Interlivros Edicoes Ltda., Rua Comandante Coelho 1085, CEP 21250, Rio de Janeiro, Brazil; and in Greek by Paschalidis Medical Publications, Athens Greece.

Surgical Clinics of North America is covered in *MEDLINE/PubMed (Index Medicus), EMBASE/Excerpta Medica, Current Contents/Clinical Medicine, Current Contents/Life Sciences, Science Citation Index,* and *ISI/BIOMED.*

Contributors

CONSULTING EDITOR

RONALD F. MARTIN, MD, FACS
Colonel (Retired), United States Army Reserve, Department of General Surgery, Pullman Regional Hospital and Clinic Network, Pullman, Washington

EDITOR

MELISSA L. KAPTANIAN, MD, FACS
Surgeon and Director, Adjunct Clinical Faculty, University of Washington School of Medicine, Adjunct Clinical Associate Professor, Pacific Northwest University of Health Sciences, Logan Health Breast Center, Physician Executive Cancer Service Line, Logan Health, Kalispell, Montana

AUTHORS

JAMES ABDO, MD
Department of Surgery, Marshfield Medical Center, Marshfield, Wisconsin

ABHISHEK CHATTERJEE, MD, MBA
Chief, Division of Plastic and Reconstructive Surgery, Tufts Medical Center; Associate Professor, Tufts University School of Medicine, Boston, Massachusetts

ALISON COOGAN, MD
Department of Surgery, Rush University Medical Center, Rush University, Chicago, Illinois

GABRIEL DE LA CRUZ KU, MD
Department of Surgery, UMass Memorial Medical Center, Worcester, Massachusetts

LYNN T. DENGEL, MD, MSc
Department of Surgery, Division of Surgical Oncology, Cancer Center, University of Virginia, Charlottesville, Virginia

AYAT ELSHERIF, MD
Division of Breast Surgery, Department of General Surgery, Cleveland Clinic, Cleveland, Ohio

LAUREN CANTER FRIEDLANDER, MD
Assistant Professor of Clinical Radiology, Division of Breast Imaging, Department of Radiology, Columbia University Irving Medical Center, New York, New York

CHRISTOPHER HOMSY, MD
Division of Plastic and Reconstructive Surgery, Tufts Medical Center, Boston, Massachusetts

HELEN M. JOHNSON, MD, IBCLC
Department of Surgery, Brody School of Medicine, East Carolina University, Greenville, North Carolina

EMILY JONES, MD
Assistant Professor, Department of Dermatology, University of Tennessee Health Science Center, Memphis, Tennessee

KARI KANSAL, MD, FACS
Associate Professor of Surgery, Chief of Breast Surgery, Department of Surgery, University of California, Irvine, Irvine, California

MANISH M. KARAMCHANDANI, MD
Department of Surgery, Tufts Medical Center, Boston, Massachusetts

LILIA LUNT, MD
Department of Surgery, Rush University Medical Center, Rush University, Chicago, Illinois

KATRINA B. MITCHELL, MD, IBCLC
Department of Surgical Oncology, Ridley-Tree Cancer Center, Sansum Clinic, Santa Barbara, California

RONA NORELIUS, MD, FAAP, FACS
Medical Director of Pediatric Surgery, Montana Children's Specialists, Logan Health, Kalispell, Montana

HOLLY ORTMAN, MD
Department of Surgery, Marshfield Medical Center, Marshfield, Wisconsin

CLAUDIA B. PEREZ, DO, MS, FACOS
Associate Professor of Surgery, Breast Surgery Oncology, Rush University Medical Center, Chicago, Illinois

SRINIDHI PULUSANI, MD
Resident, Department of Dermatology, University of Tennessee Health Science Center, Memphis, Tennessee

RACHEL E. SARGENT, MD
Department of Surgery, Los Angeles County + University of Southern California (LAC+USC) Medical Center, Department of Surgery, Keck School of Medicine of USC, University of Southern California, Los Angeles, California

STEPHEN F. SENER, MD, FACS, FSSO
Professor, Department of Surgery, Keck School of Medicine of USC, Los Angeles, California

ANNA SEYDEL, MD
Associate Professor, Director of Surgical Breast Care, Department of Surgery, Marshfield Medical Center, Marshfield, Wisconsin

HOWARD C. SNIDER, MD
Montgomery, Alabama

BRADFORD L. SOKOL, BS
Tufts University School of Medicine, Boston, Massachusetts

ALYSSA D. THROCKMORTON, MD, FACS
Clinical Assistant Professor, Department of Surgery, University of Tennessee Health Science Center, Memphis, Tennessee; Medical Director, Breast Program, Baptist Medical Group, Germantown, Tennessee

SHANNON N. TIERNEY, MD, MS, FACS
Breast Surgeon and Medical Director of Breast Program, Augusta Health Breast Surgery, Fishersville, Virginia

RACHEL TILLMAN, MD
Department of Surgery, Marshfield Medical Center, Marshfield, Wisconsin

STEPHANIE A. VALENTE, DO, FACS
Associate Professor of Surgery, Breast Surgical Oncologist, Director West Region Breast Surgery, Medical Director Fairview Breast Program, Program Director Breast Surgery Fellowship, Cleveland, Ohio

RICK D. VAVOLIZZA, MD
Department of Surgery, Division of Surgical Oncology, Cancer Center, University of Virginia, Charlottesville, Virginia

LISA WIECHMANN, MD, FACS
Division of Breast Surgery, Department of Surgery, Columbia University Irving Medical Center, New York, New York

JINGJING YU, MD
General Surgery Resident, Department of Surgery, University of California, Irvine, Irvine, California

Contents

Breast pain is a common symptom in most women during their lifetime, and many times is self-limited. Mastalgia is categorized into 3 main groups: cyclic, noncyclic and extramammary. A good history, examination and targeted imaging can help to delineate the underlying cause of mastalgia and therefore guide treatment options. Diet, medications, stress, hormonal fluctuations, and an ill-fitting bra can be contributing factors for physiologic causes of mastalgia. Breast cancer is rarely a cause but should be excluded. Reassurance, support, dietary changes, nonsteroidal anti-inflammatory drugs and occasionally hormonal medications are options to help with improving breast pain.

Lobular neoplasia (LN) is a term that describes atypical epithelial lesions originating in the terminal duct-lobular unit (TDLU) of the breast, including atypical lobular hyperplasia (ALH) and lobular carcinoma in situ (LCIS). LN is both a risk factor and nonobligate precursor to invasive breast cancer. A diagnosis of LCIS is associated with a 7-to-10-fold increased risk of breast cancer compared with the general population. When classic LN is diagnosed on a core needle biopsy (CNB), the patient may proceed with either increased screening or excisional biopsy of the lesion. Physicians should counsel patients diagnosed with LN on the risk of developing invasive carcinoma and inform them of the current screening and chemoprevention recommendations to reduce risk.

The most common manifestation of papillary breast disease is intraductal papilloma (IDP). As breast disease management becomes more refined, increasing attention has been directed at determining which IDPs require excision, and which can be monitored. This article will discuss the most common factors currently impacting personalized decision-making.

Breast imaging plays an essential role in the diagnosis and management of breast disease. From screening asymptomatic patients to evaluating clinical abnormalities on diagnostic studies, breast imaging provides critical information to the breast surgeon. Available imaging studies include those that have been proved over many years, like mammography, and those that take advantage of increasingly sophisticated technology, like breast MRI. Image-guided biopsy provides a safe means of evaluating indeterminate findings on imaging. Understanding how these tools are best used can help breast surgeons provide the best care for their patients.

There are many dermatologic conditions that can involve the skin of the breast including malignancy, infections, and inflammatory conditions. These are summarized here including presentation and management options.

The developmental phases of the breast are fluid and spread throughout prenatal, postnatal, and adolescent life. Developmental derangement during each phase can lead to disease formation. Before reaching adulthood, most abnormalities of the breast are benign in nature and can be characterized as congenital disorders, developmental disorders, or acquired disorders. Surgical intervention early in life is rarely warranted.

Nipple discharge is the third most common breast-related complaint but is rarely the presenting symptom of breast cancer. Distinguishing patients with physiologic versus pathologic nipple discharge, and treating the later according to the underlying pathologic condition is of utmost importance. Nipple discharge is categorized as lactational, physiologic, or pathologic. Physiologic nipple discharge (galactorrhea) is typically caused by hyperprolactinemia due to medications (ie, antipsychotics), pituitary tumors, and endocrine disorders. When a suspicious radiologic lesion is identified, pathologic assessment of the lesion is indicated. Patients with pathologic nipple discharge should be referred to a breast surgeon for definitive treatment and follow-up.

Cystic conditions are the most common disorder of the breast. Simple cysts are not malignant and do not require intervention. Patients with symptomatic simple cysts can undergo elective aspiration, and typical cyst fluid can be discarded. Bloody fluid should be sent for cytology. Cysts with thick walls, thick septations, or solid components have a risk of malignancy and should undergo biopsy.

Management of Mastitis, Abscess, and Fistula

Howard C. Snider

Peripheral nonlactational abscesses behave like other soft tissue abscesses and resolve with drainage and antibiotics. Subareolar abscesses tend to recur or develop fistulae between obstructed ducts and the border of the areola and are usually seen in women in their thirties who have a history of smoking or a congenitally cleft nipple. The underlying cause of subareolar abscesses and fistulae is the obstruction of terminal ducts due to keratin plugging caused by squamous metaplasia of the ducts. Successful resolution of the problem requires excision of the terminal ducts in and just below the nipple along with the correction of nipple deformity, if present.

SURGICAL CLINICS OF NORTH AMERICA

SERIES OF RELATED INTEREST

Advances in Surgery
https://www.advancessurgery.com/
Surgical Oncology Clinics
https://www.surgonc.theclinics.com/
Thoracic Surgery Clinics
http://www.thoracic.theclinics.com/

THE CLINICS ARE AVAILABLE ONLINE!
Access your subscription at:
www.theclinics.com

Foreword

Management of Benign Breast Disease

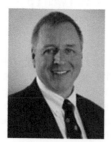

Ronald F. Martin, MD, FACS
Consulting Editor

I would submit that the term "benign disease" is oxymoronic. No disease, condition, or other pathologic process is necessarily perceived as benign—at least to the person who suffers from it. To be certain, there are diseases that have lesser or greater impacts on our longevity or quality of life than others. And perhaps once upon a time, the "malignancies" were all thought to be among worse actors compared with nonmalignant conditions. That remains true to some extent. In reality, what determines our perception of malign versus benign clinical behavior is far more related to our collective capacity ability to negate, reverse, or otherwise alter the clinical course for a patient based on our abilities and options than the underlying biology of the process. It would be challenging to imagine anyone who wants a diagnosis of a malignancy, and there are some malignant conditions I would gladly trade for some benign diagnoses.

Throughout our development of understanding of human health, malignancy and the very word "cancer" have evoked a basal fear. For much of recorded medical history that limbic fear reaction to malignancy was well deserved and in many cases still is. This primal emotion has been helpful to us in some ways. Our understandable fear of malignant conditions has motivated us to learn and develop responses in ways that our sentiments toward few other disease processes have. At present, a proposed national reaction to cancer or malignancy is being tried out as a rallying cry for united effort, suggesting that cancer treatment and eradication should be the "moonshot" of our time. Any number of advocacy groups have very successfully raised funds for the treatment of many types of cancer, in part by appealing to our collective fear of malignancy. It is difficult to find similarly successful analogues for most of the benign disorders. Perhaps some of the severe neurologic maladies or cardiac conditions or maybe some of the conditions that afflict children have had success in as much public

Surg Clin N Am 102 (2022) xiii–xiv
https://doi.org/10.1016/j.suc.2022.09.001
0039-6109/22/© 2022 Published by Elsevier Inc.

awareness and community support, but their collective efforts pale in comparison to their malignant cousins.

Our intrinsic biases toward conditions that are considered benign may also affect our perception of what medical support we require. While patients may desire to seek "specialty care" for some malignant conditions of some organs, they may be less inclined to make an extra effort for a benign process of the very same organ. Also, some organ specialty clinics may be more receptive to accommodating a patient referred for management of a malignant diagnosis than a benign one. I won't pretend to posit a "right" answer to the questions of proprieties of making referrals and accepting them—there are always many forces at play that are region, facility, and patient specific that need to be evaluated.

For those patients who suffer from a benign process of the breast, it rarely feels benign to the patient. Perhaps there is pain or discomfort. Perhaps there is concern it will have a secondary effect on a baby. Perhaps there is a concern that the process isn't benign after all. All these concerns may cause anxiety aplenty for many people. Most people do not have ready access to specialty care of every type in a timely manner. And most people want (more than anything else) timely reassurance that they are not in dire straits.

Many patients with benign breast conditions can be reassured and well treated by many different generalists and specialists if the person providing the care is reasonably well versed in the basics. At the minimum, adequate reassurance to allow the patient to follow a logical course of diagnosis and treatment can usually be achieved. Dr Kaptanian and her colleagues have put together a very informative and valuable collection of articles that will help all of us sift through the sometimes-foggy mass of information and focus on excellent basic guiding principles. I have had the distinct privilege of working directly with some of the authors who have contributed to this issue, and I can attest to their excellent clinical skill and compassion.

Just because a process is benign doesn't inherently make it easier or harder to deal with than a malignant disorder. Those who possess an excellent knowledge base combined with good clinical skill and dedication are best suited to provide the best outcomes for patients with benign or malignant disorders. That is what our patients and families desire from us, and it is what we should strive to deliver. I hope this collection of articles makes it easier for all of us to achieve that goal.

Ronald F. Martin, MD, FACS
Colonel (retired), United States Army Reserve
Department of General Surgery
Pullman Surgical Associates
Pullman Regional Hospital and Clinic Network
825 Southeast Bishop Boulevard, Suite 130
Pullman, WA 99163, USA

E-mail address:
rfmcescna@gmail.com

Preface

Management of Benign Breast Disease

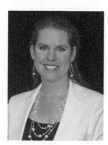

Melissa L. Kaptanian, MD, FACS
Editor

Breast cancer is thankfully not the most common breast complaint that brings a woman to the attention of a surgeon. Although 12% of American women will be diagnosed with breast cancer in their lifetime, more than 70% will be affected by a benign breast disease ranging from mastalgia to breast cysts to nipple discharge, among others. Breast cancer is often treated by a team of specialists who all benefit from the ability to present these patients at a multidisciplinary breast conference, but there is no equivalent structure for the treatment of benign diseases. Often, evaluation and management fall entirely to the surgeon.

This issue of *Surgical Clinics* is intended for that surgeon. The contributors are from diverse backgrounds, including high-volume surgeons from community medical centers and professors at academic institutions. Some of their contributions overlap and even provide different viewpoints on the same issues. This is by design. Here is the conversation we all wish we could have with colleagues on often challenging cases of benign breast diseases, their diagnosis, and management. This is the multidisciplinary tumor board for the times when there is no tumor.

My sincere thanks to the authors who rose to the challenge of having this conversation in print. Their care in making this publication educational, readable, and dare I say

Surg Clin N Am 102 (2022) xv–xvi
https://doi.org/10.1016/j.suc.2022.07.019
0039-6109/22/© 2022 Published by Elsevier Inc.

surgical.theclinics.com

even enjoyable is so appreciated. I hope that the reader finds their insights and advice useful in caring for their patients who present with these benign breast diseases.

Melissa L. Kaptanian, MD, FACS
Logan Health Breast Center
Physician Executive Cancer Service Line
Logan Health
310 Sunnyview Lane
Kalispell, MT 59901, USA

E-mail address:
mkaptanian@logan.org

Management of Mastalgia

Ayat ElSherif, MD, Stephanie A. Valente, DO*

KEYWORDS

- Mastalgia • Breast pain • Cyclic pain • Noncyclic • Mastodynia
- Extramammary pain • Tamoxifen • Danazol

KEY POINTS

- Patients with new, persistent focal breast pain should undergo a history, examination, and targeted imaging to determine the underlying cause.
- Most breast pain is self-limited and will resolve spontaneously over time and therefore reassurance and support is the first step in initial treatment.
- Some women experience prolonged and debilitating breast pain. In these cases evaluating stress factors, modifying diet, and nonsteroidal anti-inflammatory drugs can be useful.
- Occasionally hormonal medications can be used short-term at the lowest possible dose to treat mastalgia.

INTRODUCTION

Mastalgia is a term describing breast pain in one or both breasts. It is the most common breast complaint experienced in 70% of women of childbearing age.[1,2] The pain is usually described as a dull aching discomfort and sometimes as heaviness or burning pain that could be unilateral or bilateral. The extent to which mastalgia disrupts the patient's normal lifestyle in terms of sleep, work, and intimacy provides a useful assessment of severity. Breast pain can be severe enough in 10% of women that it significantly interferes with a woman's activities of daily living.[3,4] Importantly, isolated breast pain is a rare symptom of breast cancer.[5] A recent study showed that the incidence of breast malignancy in women who underwent mammogram for breast pain was 1.8%.[6] The etiology of mastalgia has been attributed to many causes. Classification of mastalgia is useful in determining the cause and ultimately the optimal plan of treatment. There are 3 main categories of breast pain, which include structural/extramammary pain (chest wall causes), cyclical mastalgia (related to menstrual cycle), or noncyclical mastalgia (not related to menstrual cycle).[7] A good breast history

Division of Breast Surgery, Department of General Surgery, Cleveland Clinic, 9500 Euclid Ave, Cleveland, OH 44195, USA
* Corresponding author.
E-mail address: Valents3@ccf.org

and examination can help the clinician identify the origin. **Fig. 1** demonstrates the management approach for mastalgia and will be reviewed in the "Management of physiologic mastalgia" section.

Examination and Workup

History
A thorough history of the pain is the first step to identify the differential of mastalgia and guide the next step in workup (**Table 1**). History should include obtaining information regarding the site, severity, duration, nature of pain, its relationship to the menstrual cycle, and any associated relieving or exacerbating factors.[8] The length of time the patient has been having pain is important, as well as review of what the patient has previously done to treat the pain. Evaluating if the pain is constant, worse at certain times of the day than others, wakes the patient up from sleep at night, or is in relation to menstrual cycle is important to discern. Review of whether patients have a normal menstrual cycle, are perimenopausal, take birth control pills or other hormonal supplements or bioidenticals is necessary history to obtain. Discussing stress is important because increased stress can play a role in breast pain. Reviewing any recent history of trauma to the breast or chest wall as asking if the patient performs any repetitive movements to the musculoskeletal system in that area (recent new exercise regimen, gardening, and so forth) can aid in identifying underlying causes. A family history of breast cancer should be obtained. A pregnancy test should be performed if history confers this possibility.[9] Medications, especially addition of new medications should be reviewed.[8]

Examination
Bilateral breast and lymph node examination should be directed primarily to exclude the presence of any masses. The patient should be examined for chest wall tenderness to exclude extramammary pain, and the breast should be gently manipulated to palpate underlying chest wall and position changes such as the patient examined in lateral semirecumbent position can be helpful.[10,11] Palpation to determine if the pain is reproducible or isolated to a certain area of the breast is helpful. Talking with

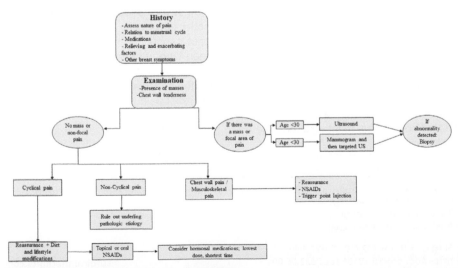

Fig. 1. Algorithm of management of mastalgia.

Table 1
Pain description at different types of mastalgia

	Cyclical Mastalgia	Noncyclical Mastalgia	Extramammary Pain
Site	Bilateral	Unilateral	Reproducible by palpation of trigger points
Relation to menstrual cycle	Related to menstrual cycle (increases 2 wk before menses)	Not related to menstrual cycle	Not related to menstrual cycle, reproducible by activity
Character	Dull, diffuse, shooting, stabbing, heaviness, aching, throbbing pain	Localized, constant or intermittent burning pain	Located at the lateral or medial side of the breast

the patient during the breast examination helps to take their mind of the examination can be helpful to physician to determine the degree of pain in relation to symptom complaints.

Anatomy
The breast receives sensory innervation from the anterior and lateral cutaneous branches of intercostal nerves as well as supraclavicular nerves. These nerves originate from T2 to T5 intercostal nerves.[12] The nipple areola complex (NAC) is supplied by the anterior and lateral cutaneous branches arising from T3 to T4. Any irritation to these nerves can lead to a referred pain that could be felt in the breast tissue or the nipple. Some women may suffer a shooting pain traveling up to the nipple; this pain is due to the irritation of a T4 branch that penetrates the deep surface of the breast before running up toward the nipple.[11]

Imaging
A woman with any new or focal symptoms should be assessed radiologically. Early breast abscess versus cyst may be difficult to determine on examination alone and ultrasound in these cases is useful. An ultrasound as first imaging modality should be performed in patients aged younger than 30 years, and mammogram followed by targeted ultrasound should be performed for patients aged 30 years or older.[13] Any suspicious mass or abnormality requires a core needle biopsy.[14,15] In some cases, breast imaging is done for reassurance to alleviate the sense of anxiety with the negative results.[16]

STRUCTURAL AND EXTRAMAMMARY CAUSES OF BREAST PAIN

First, it is important for a clinician to assess the structural components of the breast and chest wall. A large breast cup size is considered one of the anatomic and extrinsic factors for the development of breast pain.[5] The weight of the breast has been hypothesized to cause breast discomfort by the resultant strain on the suspensory ligaments.[17] Women with a large breast cup size are more likely to experience breast pain after participating in sports activities, especially with ill-fitted nonsupportive bras.[18] Determining how a women feels about bras is important. For example, asking if she wears one consistently, intermittently, or not at all can be helpful. Large breasts can benefit from the support of a well-fitted bra and could be an easy solution to breast pain. It is estimated that 70% to 90% of women wear a wrong size bra and approximately 25% of women have never been measured for a cup size before.[19] Studies have shown that breast pain is related to the actual breast cup size rather than the bra band size.[18,20-22] Another study showed that ill-fitted bra creates chaffing and shoulder strap discomfort.[20] Seventy-five percent of the breast weight should be supported by the back strap.[23] Proper cup size and well-fitted bra provide breast pain improvement in 75% to 85% of women.[23,24] A recent study compared the effect of wearing a sports bra versus receiving danazol for breast pain; women who wore a sports bra experienced higher pain relief after 12 weeks than those who received danazol (85% vs 58%). Additionally, wearing a sports bra comes with no side effects, whereas 42% of women who received danazol suffered side effects.[24] The "best-fit" bra size method was recently introduced; this method is based on professional bra fitting criteria.[25] The discrepancies in cup size measurements between retail companies can lead to inconsistent bra size and subject women to breast discomfort, and therefore, a bra-sizing measurement can be offered to patients at breast clinics.[17]

Some women with bilateral diffuse breast pain and macromastia may have structural pain related to breast size that does not improve with bra support. Breast pain that causes headaches, back pain, and an examination showing shoulder bra strap grooves in a macromastia patient are signs that the weight of their breast size itself is causing the pain. These patients would benefit from a formal breast reduction to alleviate pain and consultation to a plastic/reconstructive surgeon to discuss this possibility is recommended.

Extramammary pain refers to the breast pain originating outside of the breast tissue; most commonly presenting as referred pain originating from the chest wall, heart, lung, or esophagus.[2] A thorough history can help rule out cardiac causes of referred chest pain. Patients with a recent hard or constant cough many also experience chest wall and referred breast pain, as well as those with gastroesophageal reflux disease or shoulder/bursitis issues. At times, electrocardiogram, chest X-ray, chest computed tomographic scan, shoulder X-ray or esophagogastroduodenoscopy may be helpful for diagnosing these causes. Musculoskeletal wall pain is more common in this setting and characterized by pain described as unilateral and reproducible by activity or palpation of chest wall trigger points. It is almost always felt on the very lateral or medial side (costochondral junction) of the breast.[11,26]

Postmenopausal women who are not on hormone replacement therapy or have a known arthritis are more likely to experience a musculoskeletal pain rather than a true mastalgia.[11] The management of extramammary breast pain requires the exclusion of true breast pain by clinical assessment and imaging.[10,11] All patients presenting with a breast pain should undergo a complete breast examination while sitting and lying on each side to allow the breast to fall away from the chest wall to palpate the underlying muscles and ribs. One of the most effective methods is to allow the patient herself to locate the point of maximal tenderness on the chest wall rather than the true breast tissue.[11] Examination of the back and dermatome patterns of the chest wall are also important, to rule other findings such as herpes zoster. The evaluation of reproducible trigger points along the medial area of the scapula on the back can help identify referred musculoskeletal pain caused by scapulothoracic bursitis.[27] For the treatment of localized trigger point pain, infiltrating the tender point with 4.5 cc xylocaine 1%, 4.5 cc bupivacaine 0.5%, or 40 mg methylprednisolone can provide long-term improvement. Repeated injections after 4 to 6 weeks can be performed to offer improved pain control.[7,11,27]

Nonsteroidal anti-inflammatory drugs (NSAIDs) and modifying any exacerbating lifestyle behaviors are crucial.[10] The use of topical NSAIDs is recommended in these cases because they act locally on the tissue where they are applied and have fewer gastrointestinal side effects.[11]

CYCLIC MASTALGIA

Cystic mastalgia is breast pain that has a temporal relation to menstrual cycle; specifically the hormonal stimulation of the breast tissue that occurs at the end of luteal phase.[28] It accounts for 67% of patients with true mastalgia who are aged 30 to 40 years.[7,29] Pain usually occurs 1 week before the start of menstruation, and the pain intensity starts to decrease by the first day of menstruation and subsides within the next few days.[11] Cyclical breast pain is usually associated with breast swelling, lumpiness, tenderness, and nodularity (also termed fibrocystic changes).[2,11] The patient describes the pain as diffuse, dull, burning, or aching that might radiate to the axilla and arm in a sharp shooting sensation due to the breast glandular association with the intercostobrachial nerve in that area.[5] Pain is usually bilateral, however, pain intensity might be higher in one side than the other.[5] The condition might be exacerbated in women receiving hormonal therapy and sometimes just before menopause ensues.[11,30] Cyclical mastalgia typically resolves spontaneously in most patients over time.[31] Cyclical mastalgia improves after menopause in 42% of patients.[30]

Hormonal Causes

Several hormonal abnormalities have been attributed to cause mastalgia, which will be reviewed here. These abnormalities included excess estrogen,[32] progesterone deficiencies,[33] discrepancies in progestin/estrogen ratio,[34] receptor sensitivity variations,[35] hyperprolactinemia,[36] water retention,[37] abnormalities in follicle-stimulating hormone and luteinizing hormone secretion,[38] and low androgens.[39]

Studies have shown that estrogen levels interestingly were similar in patients with mastalgia versus asymptomatic controls.[40–44] Studies evaluating progesterone levels have produced discrepant results with some showing a significantly low luteal progesterone level among the mastalgia patients,[34,45,46] whereas other studies refuted this finding.[42,43,47,48] Regarding hyperprolactinemia, several studies have reported a significantly higher level of prolactin and hyperresponsiveness of prolactin to thyrotropin-releasing hormone stimulation among mastalgia patients.[38,49,50] Additionally, several studies have addressed the possibility of water retention in mastalgia patients and concluded that there is no correlation between breast pain and total body water between mastalgia patients and controls.[37,38] This observation supports no benefit to the use of diuretics or sodium restriction in mastalgia patients.[51]

Nonhormonal Causes

Dietary habits and lifestyle are also 2 major hypotheses of the factors in the pathophysiology of mastalgia. For patients with breast pain, discussion regarding keeping a food diary, avoiding trigger foods, and improving a healthy diet can be helpful. Patients should be reassured that this improvement may take 6 to 8 weeks to notice. Some theories regarding breast pain causes and therefore interventions are discussed below.

Methylxanthines are naturally occurring substances that are found in many food products such as coffee, tea, and chocolate. Methylxanthines are implicated as a possible cause of mastalgia because they increase cyclic adenosine monophosphate (cAMP) levels by inhibiting the enzyme responsible for the hydrolysis of cAMP, which has a role in the increased production of catecholamines. Additionally stress, nicotine, and tyramine (found in red wine, for example) can increase catecholamine levels. Catecholamines in turn can stimulate cellular proliferation and cause a hypersensitivity of the breast tissue thereby creating fibrocystic breast changes and resultant mastalgia.[52–54] Randomized clinical trial (RCTs), which investigated the efficacy of methylxanthine abstinence, demonstrated breast pain symptom resolution after

8 weeks,[54–56] whereas other studies showed no benefit after abstinence for 6 months.[57–59]

Soy milk is rich in genistein and isoflavones, which are phytoestrogens that bind to estrogen receptors and block estrogen binding, thus potentially relieving mastalgia.[60,61] In a trial that investigated the use of soy milk versus cow milk, 56% of the soy-milk group reported symptom relief versus 10% of the control cow-milk group. The challenge encountered with the use of soy milk was the unpopular taste of soy milk for many patients.[62]

Lipid and Essential Fatty Acids

A high-fat diet or abnormal lipid metabolism has been hypothesized to be a cause of mastalgia. This is based on the theory that increased lipid levels can have similar clinical effects as increased endogenous estrogen levels because estrogen is a steroid hormone, which is essentially synthesized from lipid.[11,63,64] Additionally, the increased saturated fat levels interfere with the formation of gamma-linolenic acid (GLA) by inhibiting the desaturation of linoleic acid, which in turn renders the breast tissue hypersensitive to estrogen.[35,65] Studies have found an elevation in high-density lipoproteins among mastalgia patients, and symptom relief occurred in these patients with the normalization of high-density and low-density lipoprotein levels.[66,67] Interestingly, one study evaluated a reduction in dietary fat intake (<15% of total calories) and found that patients on a low-fat diet had significant reduction in breast swelling and tenderness at 6 months compared with patients on placebo.[64]

Another theory is that women with breast pain have lower levels of essential fatty acids. Essential fatty acids are important for the normal function of the cell membrane receptors of the breast. Deficiency of essential fatty acids could create a supersensitive state and perpetuate the inflammatory component of mastalgia.[68] Additionally, essential fatty acids inhibit prostaglandin production and therefore have anti-inflammatory effects.[35,68]

Vitamins

Studies reporting on the efficacy of vitamin E on mastalgia relief have showed inconsistent results.[69–71] It has been shown that there was no superior benefit of vitamin E over placebo in the management of benign breast pain, although 40% of patients reported some improvement, it was not clinically significant.[71] Similarly, vitamin B1 and B6 did not significantly improve cyclical mastalgia.[72–75] Non-RCTs showed that the use of vitamin A in mastalgia patients lead to symptom improvement but Vitamin A was associated with toxic side effects such as skin and mucosal dryness, owing to the high daily dose needed.[76,77]

Iodine

It has been hypothesized that an iodine-deficient diet renders the breast tissue more sensitive to estrogen.[78] Iodine was found to have extrathryoid actions especially on the breast, specifically the epithelium of terminal intralobular ducts.[79] A few studies have investigated the effect of prescribing molecular iodine to mastalgia patients and have shown to be beneficial for breast pain. Molecular iodine has no effect on the thyroid, so there are no side effects, only the benefits of breast pain relief.[78,80] A study reported that more than 50% of women who took a daily iodine supplement of 6 mg showed resolution of breast pain at 6 months.[80] A novel iodine formulation, IoGen, which generates molecular iodine by the action of gastric juice, was also examined and a significant improvement was noted in 50% of mastalgia patients after 6 months.[80]

Smoking

An observational study showed that smoking women are more likely to suffer from breast pain than nonsmokers.[4] The mechanism by which smoking causes mastalgia remains unclear. It has been hypothesized that smoking interrupts the production of endogenous estrogen, as smoking women were found to have low estrogen levels and experienced early menopause; however, this contradicts the common knowledge that mastalgia is caused by excess estrogen.[32,81,82]

Activity

Breast pain is more common in women with a sedentary lifestyle and low activity levels.[20,22]

Psychological

Despite the growing theories that mastalgia patients can be associated with a psychosomatic disorder, due to some cases of no clear organic cause to the pain, this association was disputed.[83] Notably, the control group scored higher for psychoneurosis than the mastalgia group.[83] However, patients with severe refractory mastalgia were noted to have a higher level of depression and anxiety.[84] It was even reported that the level of anxiety and depression in the mastalgia patients is comparable to that of patients with breast cancer at the morning of their surgery.[85] These mood disorders were more likely to be present in patients with severe mastalgia rather than nonsevere mastalgia.[85,86] In the light of these potential disorders, patients with severe mastalgia without an underlying cause and nonresponsive to conservative measures should be screened and proper psychological support should be provided if indicated.[86]

NONCYCLIC MASTALGIA

Noncyclic mastalgia is breast pain that is nonhormonal and unrelated to menstrual cycle. It accounts for one-third of the patients referred to breast clinic.[8] Pain is usually described as constant or intermittent localized burning pain. It is almost always unilateral and confined to one quadrant.[87] It affects perimenopausal women typically in their 40s and 50s.[13,28] Unlike cyclical pain, it does not have a precipitating factor and has a shorter duration with a spontaneous resolution without treatment in 50% of the cases.[9,30] However, pain might exacerbate without an apparent underlying cause and become more difficult to treat.[3,5]

Noncyclical pain can be inflammatory, vascular, or neoplastic in nature. There are several causes for this type of pain, which include a pendulous breast, stretching of Cooper's ligaments, breast cysts, traumatic fat necrosis, mastitis (lactational or nonlactational), breast abscess, duct ectasia, diabetic mastopathy, superficial thrombophlebitis (Mondor disease) or previous breast surgery.[2,8,29] Breast imaging can identify many of these causes that can be improved with targeted treatment.

MANAGEMENT OF PHYSIOLOGIC MASTALGIA
Conservative and Supportive Treatment

Reassurance and daily pain charting
The first step in managing mastalgia is reassurance.[51] Reassuring patients that their symptoms are not related to cancer or any serious disease will alleviate their anxiety.[8,28] Reassurance was found to be sufficient in 85% of patients with mild symptoms, 70% in moderate cases, and 52% in severe cases.[88] Reassurance is especially recommended in patients who exhibit mood disorders such as depression

and anxiety.[88] Incorporating a daily activity provides symptoms relief because it decreases estrogen levels.[2] Relaxation therapy has some potential in pain relief with 61% of women showing substantial pain relief in comparison to 25% in the control group as well as improvement in pain-free duration.[89] Wearing a well-fitted bra or sports bra that provides support and reduces pressure on suspensory ligaments of the breast was proven to be significantly efficient in pain relief.[90] Applying hot and cold compresses to the breast especially at nighttime showed some improvement.[2]

Asking the patient to note the severity of pain in the daily chart using the visual analog scale (VAS) is beneficial in providing reliable data about severity and duration of pain and its association to the menstrual cycle.[29,31] A VAS score of 3 or greater is considered to be significantly associated with severe pain and requiring therapy.[91] **Fig. 2** shows the VAS. Having the patient keep a daily pain and dietary log will be helpful in determining the cause in unknown cases as well of what type of intervention may be best.

Diet and lifestyle modifications
A low-fat diet (<15% fat/d) has been shown to have some beneficial effects in reducing pain.[66,67] Reducing food containing methylxanthines or increasing food rich in vitamins (A, B1, B6, E) did not show superior benefits when compared with giving placebo but may be discussed with patients as dietary change options.

Over-the-Counter Medications and Supplements

Oral and topical analgesics
NSAIDs are effective for the treatment of mastalgia in approximately 80% of patients.[29] The use of topical forms is recommended because it has fewer side effects than systemic forms.[92] The stronger types of topical NSAIDs such as diclofenac and piroxicam (such as aspercreame or voltaren gel) are more effective than weaker types such as ibuprofen.[73,92] Diclofenac gel to the breast every 8 hours demonstrated decreased pain noticed at 15 days.[92] Use of stronger agents, either topical or systemic, can be helpful to patients with both cyclical and noncyclical breast pain.[92–94] Opiates are not recommended for the treatment of physiologic breast pain.

Alternative therapies
Evening Primrose oil (EPO) and its active form, GLA, have been used for the treatment of mastalgia due to the fact that mastalgia patients have essential fatty acid

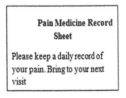
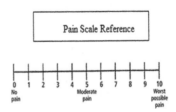

Fig. 2. Visual analog pain scale.

deficiency.[35,95,96] However, most of the large multicentric trials reported improvement in breast pain but there was no significant difference between the EPO group and the placebo group.[97–100] These studies refute the efficacy of EPO and GLA for mastalgia. For patients interested in trialing alternative therapies, the recommendation is to either use EPO ointment topically applied to the breast or as an oral supplement of up to 1 g per day because it has minimal side effects and may be effective in some women. Additionally, Flaxseed 25 mg daily and Chasteberry (Vitex angus) 3.2 to 4.8 mg supplementation has been evaluated as natural supplements, which have shown to be helpful to significantly reduce breast pain during a 2 month period and could be considered.[101] Chasteberry or Angus castus, a fruit extract, was shown to be well tolerated and lead to an improvement of pain score on the VAS.[102,103] Other herbs such as ginseng should be avoided because some studies reported that mastalgia is common complaint in women consuming ginseng.[104,105]

Rarely, breast pain significantly inhibits ones daily life activities and additional therapies need to be considered. In this situation, the balance the breast pain complaints versus the side effects of treatment needs to be evaluated and discussed with the focus being on treatment for the shortest amount of time that gives benefit with the understanding that trial of stopping treatment may result in the return of breast pain symptoms.

Hormonal Treatments

Tamoxifen

Tamoxifen is a selective estrogen receptor modulator (SERM) because it carries estrogen agonist effects on uterus and bones but antiestrogen effect on the breast.[106] It is widely used in the treatment of breast cancer. Tamoxifen 20 mg was found to be associated with mastalgia improvement in 71% of cases.[107] However, a wide spectrum of menopausal side effects such as hot flashes, sweating, fatigue, nausea, menstrual irregularities, weight gain, bloating, and vaginal dryness were reported.[108] The efficacy of low dose tamoxifen 10 mg was compared with 20 mg dose, higher doses were not more effective but were associated with higher risk of side effects.[109,110] Side effects were reported in 65% of 20 mg group and 20% in the 10 mg group.[109] Moreover, administering tamoxifen only during the luteal phase of the menstrual cycle was associated with fewer side effects and with pain improvement in 85% of women regardless of the dose given.[111]

A recent meta-analysis that compared the efficacy of tamoxifen, bromocriptine, danazol, and placebo showed that tamoxifen is the most effective with the lower side effects.[98] However, tamoxifen is associated with some serious side effects such as endometrial carcinoma and high risk of thromboembolic disease, especially in smokers.[112,113]

A newer generation SERM, toremifene, was compared with tamoxifen and showed that toremifene had comparable therapeutic effects to tamoxifen with fewer side effects.[82] Toremifene was associated with mastalgia improvement in 64% of patients.[114]

Topical gel containing a potent tamoxifen metabolite, afimoxifene has been examined for the management of mastalgia. Topical afimoxifene 4 mg showed a significant symptom relief compared with placebo. The use of such topical form was not associated with side effects because it has 1000-fold lower serum level compared with oral forms.[115]

There are set of precautions to consider when using tamoxifen for mastalgia:

(a) Patient must be informed that tamoxifen is given for mastalgia not cancer.[116]

(b) Low dose (10 mg) given during the luteal phase only should be used to avoid side effects.[11,111]

(c) Tamoxifen is contraindicated in patients with history of thromboembolic disease.[51]

(d) Tamoxifen should be stopped after 3 months if there is no effect.[2,116]

(e) The regimen (10 mg) should be reviewed after 3 months and titrated according to the severity of pain to either reducing the dose to every other day or increasing the dose to 20 mg.[110]

Progesterone (topical, oral, vaginal)

The different forms of progesterone have been studied for the management of mastalgia. Sixty-six to 80% of the patients reported significant pain improvement on micronized progesterone.[117,118] However, hormonal treatment should not be taken for more than 6 months owing to the risk of side effects as nausea, vomiting, weight gain, and metrorrhagia.[29] Oral medroxyprogesterone is not effective against mastalgia and its therapeutic effect was not superior over placebo in cyclical mastalgia.[119]

Danazol

Danazol is a testosterone derivative, which has an antigonadotrophin actions and mild androgenic effects.[120,121] It is the only drug approved by the Food and Drug Administration for the treatment of mastalgia. Danazol 200 mg has been proven to be efficient in symptom resolution as early as in 4 weeks.[122] The rate of noncompliance is high owing to the intolerable androgenic side effects as acne, voice changes, weight gain, hirsutism, hot flushes, menstrual irregularities, depression, headache, and dyspareunia.[123] Women at child-bearing age should be advised to take a nonhormonal contraceptive while taking danazol. Danazol is contraindicated in women with thromboembolic disease and pregnant women due to teratogenicity.[5] In the light of these wide spectrum of side effects, danazol should be reserved for women with severe mastalgia who failed to respond to 3 to 6 months of tamoxifen and should be given in the luteal phase only.[124,125]

Gestrinone

Gestrinone, an androgen derivative, is a synthetic steroid similar to danazol but does not require contraception. Gestrinone was found to improve mastalgia in 55% of patients in 3 months of use; however, owing to the antiestrogen and antiprogesterone effects, 41% of women suffered side effects as hirsutism, acne, menstrual irregularities, and reduced breast size.[126,127] Low doses have fewer side effects.

Bromocriptine

Hyperprolactinemia is one of the hormonal causes of mastalgia.[36] This lead to examining the effect of dopaminergic agonists such as bromocriptine in relieving mastalgia. Bromocriptine is an ergot alkaloid that suppresses prolactin secretion. Studies reported that lowering prolactin by the use of bromocriptine was associated with a significant symptom improvement specifically in the cyclical mastalgia patients but not in the noncyclical mastalgia patients.[75,128,129] Relief of mastalgia was reported in 65% and side effects occurred in 45% of patients with 11% discontinuation rate. Side effects reported were nausea, headaches, and dizziness due to hypotension.[128] Studies have shown that serious side effects as seizure, stroke, and death might occur during bromocriptine use, which limited its indications.[130] Cabergoline, a newer generation, traditionally used to treat high prolactin levels is a long-lasting dopamine agonist that was found to be as effective as bromocriptine with fewer side effects and no tendency to serious side effects.[131]

When comparing bromocriptine efficacy to the danazol, higher response rate was reported with danazol.[75] Owing to the associated side effects, bromocriptine use is limited and no longer recommended except in cases where danazol is contraindicated as in women with thromboembolic diseases.[110]

Holistic Medicine

Acupuncture

Alternative therapies such as inserting acupuncture needles at the inner side of the arm in the pressure point to relief mastalgia have been documented.[132,133] Overall, 67% of women who underwent acupuncture reported significant symptom improvement.[133] In some women, pain might be localized to a specific point; massaging this tender point can also lead to pain relief in 60% of patients.[134] Further studies are needed for the use of kinesiology and holistic medicine in the management of mastalgia.

RECOMMENDATIONS

- A thorough history and careful examination can differentiate between true mastalgia and extramammary pain.
- Breast imaging should be performed for new complains of breast pain, especially focal pain in the breast.
- Reassurance is the mainstay of treatment for most of cyclical mastalgia patients without an underlying cause.
- Low-fat diet with active lifestyle and the use of well-fitting bra provide symptom relief for true mastalgia patients.
- NSAIDs are considered first-line treatment of mastalgia especially topical forms such as diclofenac and piroxicams.
- Tamoxifen or danazol should be considered as second-line treatment after reassurance and simple analgesics failure.
- Surgery should not be considered in the management of mastalgia.

FUNDING

No funding. Dr. Valente is a consultat/ speaker for Impedimed, Merit Medical, AxoGen and Pacira

DISCLOSURE

The authors have nothing to disclose.

CLINICS CARE POINTS

- Breast pain requires a good history physical to determine the underlying cause, with directed imaging as needed.
- Breast pain can be categorized into noncyclical, cyclical, and extramammary/structural.
- Most patients with physiologic breast pain can be managed with reassurance, dietary modifications, over-the-counter topical medications and time.
- Occasionally, physiologic breast pain can be severe and consideration for additional therapies should be discussed.

REFERENCES

1. Dixon JM, Thomas J. 1 Symptoms, assessment, and guidelines for referral. ABC Breast Dis 2012;1.
2. Tahir MT, Shamsudeen S. Mastalgia. InStatPearls [Internet] 2021 Feb 14. StatPearls Publishing.35. D.F. Horrobin (Ed.), Omega-6 Essential Fatty Acids: Pathophysiology and Roles in Clinical Medicine, Wiley-Liss, New York (1990), pp. 20-5384. Yilmaz ED, Deveci E, Kadioglu H, et al. Anxiety and depression levels and personality traits of mastalgia patients. J Psychiatr. 2014; 17–118
3. Mansel R, Webster DJ, Sweetland H. Chapter 8: Breast pain and nodularity. Benign Disorders and Diseases of the Breast. Elsevier; 2009. p. 107–39.
4. Ader D, South-Paul J, Adera T, et al. Cyclical mastalgia: prevalence and associated health and behavioral factors. J Psychosomatic Obstet Gynecol 2001; 22(2):71–6.
5. Sasaki J, Geletzke A, Kass RB, Klimberg SV, Copeland EM, Bland KI, et al. Etiology and management of benign breast disease. The Breast, . The Breast (5th Edition). Elsevier; 2018. p. 79–92.
6. Noroozian M, Stein LF, Gaetke-Udager K, et al. Long-term clinical outcomes in women with breast pain in the absence of additional clinical findings: mammography remains indicated. Breast Cancer Res Treat 2015;149(2):417–24.
7. Maddox P, Harrison B, Mansel R, et al. Non-cyclical mastalgia: an improved classification and treatment. J Br Surg 1989;76(9):901–4.
8. Evaluation and management of breast pain.. In: Smith RL, Pruthi S, Fitzpatrick LA, editors. Mayo Clinic Proceedings79. Elsevier; 2004. p. 353–72.
9. Gumm R, Cunnick G, Mokbel K. Evidence for the management of mastalgia. Curr Med Res Opin 2004;20(5):681–4.
10. Hubbard TJ, Sharma A, Ferguson DJ. Breast pain: assessment, management, and referral criteria. Br J Gen Pract 2020;70(697):419–20.
11. Iddon J, Dixon JM. Mastalgia. Bmj 2013;347.
12. Woodworth GE, Ivie RMJ, Nelson SM, et al. Perioperative Breast Analgesia: A Qualitative Review of Anatomy and Regional Techniques. Reg Anesth pain Med 2017;42(5):609–31.
13. Leung JW, Kornguth PJ, Gotway MB. Utility of targeted sonography in the evaluation of focal breast pain. J Ultrasound Med 2002;21(5):521–6.
14. Harper AP, Kelly-Fry E, Noe JS. Ultrasound breast imaging-the method of choice for examining the young patient. Ultrasound Med Biol 1981;7(3):231–7.
15. Howard MB, Battaglia T, Prout M, et al. The effect of imaging on the clinical management of breast pain. J Gen Intern Med 2012;27(7):817–24.
16. Zarei F, Pishdad P, Hatami M, et al. Can breast ultrasound reduce patient's level of anxiety and pain? Ultrasound 2017;25(2):92–7.
17. Hafiz SP, Barnes NL, Kirwan CC. Clinical management of idiopathic mastalgia: a systematic review. J Prim Health Care 2018;10(4):312–23.
18. Brown N, White J, Brasher A, et al. The experience of breast pain (mastalgia) in female runners of the 2012 London Marathon and its effect on exercise behaviour. Br J Sports Med 2014;48(4):320–5.
19. Robb GL, Hortobagyi GN. Advanced therapy of breast disease. PMPH-USA; 2004.
20. Brown N, White J, Brasher A, et al. An investigation into breast support and sports bra use in female runners of the 2012 London Marathon. J Sports Sci 2014;32(9):801–9.

21. Burnett E, White J, Scurr J. The Influence of the breast on physical activity participation in females. J Phys Activity Health 2015;12(4).
22. Brown N, Burnett E, Scurr J. Is breast pain greater in active females compared to the general population in the UK? Breast J 2016;22(2):194–201.
23. Wilson M, Sellwood R. Therapeutic value of a supporting brassiere in mastodynia. Br Med J 1976;2(6027):90.
24. Hadi MSA. Sports brassiere: is it a solution for mastalgia? Breast J 2000;6(6): 407–9.
25. White J, Scurr J. Evaluation of professional bra fitting criteria for bra selection and fitting in the UK. Ergonomics 2012;55(6):704–11.
26. Ambramson D. Lateral extra mammary pain syndrome. Breast (Edinburgh, Scotland) 1980;6:2–5.
27. Boneti C, Arentz C, Klimberg VS. Scapulothoracic bursitis as a significant cause of breast and chest wall pain: underrecognized and undertreated. Ann Surg Oncol 2010;17(3):321–4.
28. Wisbey J, Mansel R, Pye J, et al. Natural history of breast pain. Lancet 1983; 322(8351):672–4.
29. Kataria K, Dhar A, Srivastava A, et al. A systematic review of current understanding and management of mastalgia. Indian J Surg 2014;76(3):217–22.
30. Davies E, Gateley C, Miers M, et al. The long-term course of mastalgia. J R Soc Med 1998;91(9):462–4.
31. Kumar S, Rai R, Das V, et al. Visual analogue scale for assessing breast nodularity in non-discrete lumpy breasts: The Lucknow–Cardiff breast nodularity scale. Breast 2010;19(3):238–42.
32. Fechner RE. Benign breast disease in women on estrogen therapy. A pathologic study. Cancer 1972;29(2):273–9.
33. Mauvais-Jarvis P, Sitruk-Ware R, Kuttenn F, et al. Luteal phase insufficiency: a common pathophysiologic factor in development of benign and malignant breast diseases. Commentaries Res Breast Dis 1979;1:25–59.
34. Sitruk-Ware L, Sterkers N, Mowszowicz I, et al. Inadequate corpus luteal function in women with benign breast diseases. J Clin Endocrinol Metab 1977; 44(4):771–4.
35. Horrobin DF, editor. Omega-6 Essential Fatty Acids: Pathophysiology and Roles in Clinical Medicine. New York: Wiley-Liss; 1990. p. 20–53.
36. Cole E, Sellwood R, England P, et al. Serum prolactin concentrations in benign breast disease throughout the menstrual cycle. Eur J Cancer (1965) 1977;13(6): 597–603.
37. Preece P, Richards A, Owen G, et al. Mastalgia and total body water. Br Med J 1975;4(5995):498–500.
38. Kumar S, Mansel R, Scanlon M, et al. Altered responses of prolactin, luteinizing hormone and follicle stimulating hormone secretion to thyrotrophin releasing hormone/gonadotrophin releasing hormone stimulation in cyclical mastalgia. Br J Surg 1984;71(11):870–3.
39. Brennan M, Bulbrook R, Deshpande N, et al. Urinary and plasma androgens in benign breast disease: Possible relation to breast cancer. Lancet 1973; 301(7812):1076–9.
40. Malarkey WB, Schroeder L, Stevens V, et al. Twenty-four-hour preoperative endocrine profiles in women with benign and malignant breast disease. Cancer Res 1977;37(12):4655–9.
41. Watt-Boolsen S, Andersen A, Blichert-Toft M. Serum prolactin and oestradiol levels in women with cyclical mastalgia. Horm Metab Res 1981;13(12):700–2.

42. Walsh PV, McDicken IW, Bulbrook RD, et al. Serum oestradiol-17β and prolactin concentrations during the luteal phase in women with benign breast disease. Eur J Cancer Clin Oncol 1984;20(11):1345–51.

43. Golinger R, Krebs J, Fisher E, et al. Hormones and the pathophysiology of fibrocystic mastopathy: elevated luteinizing hormone levels. Surgery 1978;84(2): 212–5.

44. Kumar S, Mansel R, Wilson D, et al. Daily salivary progesterone levels in cyclical mastalgia patients and their controls. Br J Surg 1986;73(4):260–3.

45. Sitruk-Ware R, Sterkers N, Mauvais-Jarvis P. Benign breast disease I: hormonal investigation. Obstet Gynecol 1979;53(4):457–60.

46. Ayers JW, Gidwani GP. The "luteal breast": hormonal and sonographic investigation of benign breast disease in patients with cyclic mastalgia. Fertil sterility 1983;40(6):779–84.

47. Walsh PV, Bulbrook RD, Stell PM, et al. Serum progesterone concentration during the luteal phase in women with benign breast disease. Eur J Cancer Clin Oncol 1984;20(11):1339–43.

48. England P, Skinner L, Cottrell K, et al. Sex hormones in breast disease. J Br Surg 1975;62(10):806–9.

49. Peters F, Pickardt C, Zimmermann G, et al. PRL, TSH, and thyroid hormones in benign breast diseases. Klinische Wochenschrift 1981;59(8):403–7.

50. Rea N, Bove F, Gentile A, et al. Prolactin response to thyrotropin-releasing hormone as a guideline for cyclical mastalgia treatment. Minerva Med 1997;88(11): 479–87.

51. Rosolowich V, Saettler E, Szuck B, et al. Mastalgia J Obstet Gynaecol Can 2006; 28(1):49–57.

52. Minton JP. Dietary factors in benign breast disease. Cancer Bull 1988;40:44.

53. Bär H-P. Epinephrine-and prostaglandin-sensitive adenyl cyclase in mammary gland. Biochim Biophys Acta (BBA)-Enzymology 1973;321(1):397–406.

54. Minton JP, Abou-Issa H. Nonendocrine theories of the etiology of benign breast disease. World J Surg 1989;13(6):680–4.

55. Minton J, Foecking M, Webster D, et al. Response of fibrocystic disease to caffeine withdrawal and correlation of cyclic nucleotides with breast disease. Am J Obstet Gynecol 1979;135(1):157–8.

56. Minton J, Abou-Issa H, Reiches N, et al. Clinical and biochemical studies on methylxanthine-related fibrocystic breast disease. Surgery 1981;90(2):299–304.

57. Ernster VL, Mason L, Goodson WH, et al. Effects of caffeine-free diet on benign breast disease: a randomized trial. Surgery 1982;91(3):263–7.

58. Allen SS, Froberg DG. The effect of decreased caffeine consumption on benign proliferative breast disease: a randomized clinical trial. Surgery 1987;101(6): 720–30.

59. Parazzini F, La Vecchia C, Riundi R, et al. Methylxanthine, alcohol-free diet and fibrocystic breast disease: a factorial clinical trial. Surgery 1986;99(5):576–81.

60. Ingram D, Hickling C, West L, et al. A double-blind randomized controlled trial of isoflavones in the treatment of cyclical mastalgia. The Breast 2002;11(2):170–4.

61. Fleming R. What effect, if any, does soy protein have on breast tissue? Integr Cancer therapies 2003;2(3):225–8.

62. McFadyen I, Chetty U, Setchell K, et al. A randomized double blind-cross over trial of soya protein for the treatment of cyclical breast pain. Breast 2000;9(5): 271–6.

63. Goodwin PJ, Miller A, Del Giudice ME, et al. Elevated high-density lipoprotein cholesterol and dietary fat intake in women with cyclic mastopathy. Am J Obstet Gynecol 1998;179(2):430–7.

64. Boyd N, Shannon P, Kriukov V, et al. Effect of a low-fat high-carbohydrate diet on symptoms of cyclical mastopathy. Lancet 1988;332(8603):128–32.

65. Horrobin D. The effects of gamma-linolenic acid on breast pain and diabetic neuropathy: possible non-eicosanoid mechanisms. Prostaglandins, Leukot Essent fatty Acids 1993;48(1):101–4.

66. Rose DP, Boyar AP, Cohen C, et al. Effect of a low-fat diet on hormone levels in women with cystic breast disease. I. Serum steroids and gonadotropins. J Natl Cancer Inst 1987;78(4):623–6.

67. Sharma A, Mishra S, Salila M, et al. Cyclical mastalgia–is it a manifestation of aberration in lipid metabolism? Indian J Physiol Pharmacol 1994;38(4):267–71.

68. Goyal A, Mansel R. on behalf of the Efamast Study Group. A Randomized multi-center study of gamolenic acid (Efamast) with and without antioxidant vitamins and minerals in the management of mastalgia. Breast J 2005;11:41–7.

69. Ernster V, Goodson W 3rd, Hunt T, et al. Vitamin E and benign breast" disease": a double-blind, randomized clinical trial. Surgery 1985;97(4):490–4.

70. Meyer E, Sommers D, Reitz C, et al. Vitamin E and benign breast disease. Surgery 1990;107(5):549–51.

71. London RS, Sundaram G, Murphy L, et al. The effect of vitamin E on mammary dysplasia: a double-blind study. Obstet Gynecol 1985;65(1):104–6.

72. Smallwood J, Ah-Kye D, Taylor I. Vitamin B6 in the treatment of pre-menstrual mastalgia. Br J Clin Pract 1986;40(12):532–3.

73. McFayden I, Forrest A, Chetty U, et al. Cyclical breast pain–some observations and the difficulties in treatment. Br J Clin Pract 1992;46(3):161–4.

74. Wetzig NR. Mastalgia: a 3 year Australian study. Aust New Zealand J Surg 1994;64(5):329–31.

75. Pye J, Mansel R, Hughes L. Clinical experience of drug treatments for mastalgia. Lancet 1985;326(8451):373–7.

76. Band PR, Deschamps M, Falardeau M, et al. Treatment of benign breast disease with vitamin A. Prev Med 1984;13(5):549–54.

77. Brocq P, Stora C, Bernheim L. De l'emploi de la vitamine A dans le traitement des mastoses. Ann Endocrinol 1956;17:193–200.

78. Ghent W, Eskin B, Low D, et al. Iodine replacement in fibrocystic disease of the breast. Can J Surg J canadien de chirurgie 1993;36(5):453–60.

79. Eskin B, Krouse T, Modhera P, et al. Etiology of mammary gland pathophysiology induced by iodine deficiency. Front thyroidology 1986;2.

80. Kessler JH. The effect of supraphysiologic levels of iodine on patients with cyclic mastalgia. Breast J 2004;10(4):328–36.

81. Wang J, Zhang H, Allen RD. Overexpression of an Arabidopsis peroxisomal ascorbate peroxidase gene in tobacco increases protection against oxidative stress. Plant Cell Physiol 1999;40(7):725–32.

82. Gong C, Song E, Jia W, et al. A double-blind randomized controlled trial of toremifen therapy for mastalgia. Arch Surg 2006;141(1):43–7.

83. Preece P, Mansel R, Hughes L. Mastalgia: psychoneurosis or organic disease? Br Med J 1978;1(6104):29–30.

84. Yilmaz ED, Deveci E, Kadioglu H, et al. Anxiety and depression levels and personality traits of mastalgia patients. J Psychiatr 2014;17:118.

85. Ramirez A-J, Jarrett SR, Hamed H, Smith P, Fentiman IP, et al. Psychosocial distress associated with severe mastalgia., . Recent developments in the study of benign breast disease. Parthenon Publishing Group LTD; 1994. p. 1019–116.

86. Ramirez A-J, Jarrett S, Hamed H, et al. Psychosocial adjustment of women with mastalgia. Breast 1995;4(1):48–51.

87. Groen J-W, Grosfeld S, Bramer WM, et al. Cyclic and non-cyclic breast-pain: A systematic review on pain reduction, side effects, and quality of life for various treatments. Eur J Obstet Gynecol Reprod Biol 2017;219:74–93.

88. Barros ACS, Mottola J Jr, Ruiz CA, et al. Reassurance in the treatment of mastalgia. Breast J 1999;5(3):162–5.

89. Fox H, Walker L, Heys S, et al. Are patients with mastalgia anxious, and does relaxation therapy help? Breast 1997;6(3):138–42.

90. Ngô C, Seror J, Chabbert-Buffet N. Breast pain: Recommendations. J de gynecologie, obstetrique biologie de la Reprod 2015;44(10):938–46.

91. Wewers ME, Lowe NK. A critical review of visual analogue scales in the measurement of clinical phenomena. Res Nurs Health 1990;13(4):227–36.

92. Colak T, Ipek T, Kanik A, et al. Efficacy of topical nonsteroidal antiinflammatory drugs in mastalgia treatment. J Am Coll Surgeons 2003;196(4):525–30.

93. Irving A, Morrison S. Effectiveness of topical non-steroidal anti-inflammatory drugs in the management of breast pain. J R Coll Surgeons Edinb 1998; 43(3):158–9.

94. Kaviani A, Mehrdad N, Najafi M, et al. Comparison of naproxen with placebo for the management of noncyclical breast pain: a randomized, double-blind, controlled trial. World J Surg 2008;32(11):2464–70.

95. Gateley C, Maddox P, Pritchard G, et al. Plasma fatty acid profiles in benign breast disorders. J Br Surg 1992;79(5):407–9.

96. Gateley C, Miers M, Mansel R, et al. Drug treatments for mastalgia: 17 years experience in the Cardiff Mastalgia Clinic. J R Soc Med 1992;85(1):12.

97. Goyal A, Mansel RE. A randomized multicenter study of gamolenic acid (Efamast) with and without antioxidant vitamins and minerals in the management of mastalgia. Breast J 2005;11(1):41–7.

98. Srivastava A, Mansel R, Arvind N, et al. Evidence-based management of Mastalgia: a meta-analysis of randomised trials. The Breast 2007;16(5):503–12.

99. Blommers J, de Lange-de Klerk ES, Kuik DJ, et al. Evening primrose oil and fish oil for severe chronic astalgia: a randomized, double-blind, controlled trial. Am J Obstet Gynecol 2002;187(5):1389–94.

100. Pruthi S, Wahner-Roedler DL, Torkelson CJ, et al. Vitamin E and evening primrose oil for management of cyclical mastalgia: a randomized pilot study. Altern Med Rev 2010;15(1):59.

101. Mirghafourvand M, Mohammad-Alizadeh-Charandabi S, Ahmadpour P, et al. Effects of Vitex agnus and Flaxseed on cyclic mastalgia: A randomized controlled trial. Complement therapies Med 2016;24:90–5.

102. Schellenberg R. Treatment for the premenstrual syndrome with agnus castus fruit extract: prospective, randomised, placebo controlled study. Bmj 2001; 322(7279):134–7.

103. Halaska M, Beles P, Gorkow C, et al. Treatment of cyclical mastalgia with a solution containing a Vitex agnus castus extract: results of a placebo-controlled double-blind study. Breast 1999;8(4):175–81.

104. Dukes M. Ginseng and mastalgia. Br Med J 1978;1(6127):1621.

105. Nocerino E, Amato M, Izzo AA. The aphrodisiac and adaptogenic properties of ginseng. Fitoterapia 2000;71:S1–5.

106. Cupceancu B. Short-term tamoxifen treatment in benign breast diseases. Endocrinologie 1985;23(3):169–77.
107. Fentiman I, Brame K, Caleffi M, et al. Double-blind controlled trial of tamoxifen therapy for mastalgia. Lancet 1986;327(8476):287–8.
108. Fentiman I, Caleffi M, Hamed H, et al. Dosage and duration of tamoxifen treatment for mastalgia: a controlled trial. Br J Surg 1988;75(9):845–6.
109. Fentiman I, Caleffi M, Hamed H, et al. Studies of tamoxifen in women with mastalgia. Br J Clin Pract Suppl 1989;68:34–53.
110. Faiz O, Fentiman I. Management of breast pain. Int J Clin Pract 2000;54(4):228–32.
111. Semiglazov V. Tamoxifen therapy for cyclical mastalgia: dose randomized trial. The Breast 1997;6(4):212–3.
112. Fisher B, Dignam J, Bryant J, et al. Five versus more than five years of tamoxifen therapy for breast cancer patients with negative lymph nodes and estrogen receptor-positive tumors. JNCI: J Natl Cancer Inst 1996;88(21):1529–42.
113. Millet AV, Leal A, Dirbas FM. Clinical management of breast pain., . Breast Surgical Techniques and Interdisciplinary management. New York, NY: Springer; 2010. p. 147–53.
114. Oksa S, Luukkaala T, Mäenpää J. Toremifene for premenstrual mastalgia: a randomised, placebo-controlled crossover study. BJOG: An Int J Obstet Gynaecol 2006;113(6):713–8.
115. Mansel R, Goyal A, Nestour EL, et al. A phase II trial of Afimoxifene (4-hydroxytamoxifen gel) for cyclical mastalgia in premenopausal women. Breast Cancer Res Treat 2007;106(3):389–97.
116. Fentiman I, Powles T. Tamoxifen and benign breast problems. Lancet 1987;330(8567):1070–2.
117. Uzan S, Denis C, Pomi V, et al. Double-blind trial of promegestone (R 5020) and lynestrenol in the treatment of benign breast disease. Eur J Obstet Gynecol Reprod Biol 1992;43(3):219–27.
118. Colin C, Gaspard U, Lambotte R. Relationship of mastodynia with its endocrine environment and treatment in a double blind trial with lynestrenol. Archiv für Gynäkologie 1978;225(1):7–13.
119. Maddox PR, Harrison B, Horobin J, et al. A randomised controlled trial of medroxyprogesterone acetate in mastalgia. Ann R Coll Surg Engl 1990;72(2):71.
120. Greenblatt RB, Dmowski W, Mahesh V, et al. Clinical studies with an antigonadotropin-danazol. Fertil Sterility 1971;22(2):102–12.
121. Chambers C, Arsch R, Panerstein C. Danazol binding and translocation of steroids receptors. Am J Obstet Gynecol 1980;136:426.
122. O'Brien PS, Abukhalil I. Randomized controlled trial of the management of premenstrual syndrome and premenstrual mastalgia using luteal phase–only danazol. Am J Obstet Gynecol 1999;180(1):18–23.
123. Sutton G, O'Malley V. Treatment of cyclical mastalgia with low dose short term danazol. Br J Clin Pract 1986;40(2):68–70.
124. Asch RH, Greenblatt RB. The use of an impeded androgen—danazol—in the management of benign breast disorders. Am J Obstet Gynecol 1977;127(2):130–4.
125. Mansel R, Wisbey J, Hughes L. Controlled trial of the antigonadotropin danazol in painful nodular benign breast disease. Lancet 1982;319(8278):928–30.
126. Snyder BW, Beecham GD, Winneker RC. Studies on the mechanism of action of danazol and gestrinone (R2323) in the rat: evidence for a masked estrogen component. Fertil sterility 1989;51(4):705–10.

127. Peters F, Brandl E, Tykal P, et al. Multicentre study of gestrinone in cyclical breast pain FRIEDOLF PETERS. Lancet 1992;339(8787):205–8.
128. Mansel R, Preece P, Hughes L. A double blind trial of the prolactin inhibitor bromocriptine in painful benign breast disease. Br J Surg 1978;65(10):724–7.
129. Hinton C, Bishop H, Holliday H, et al. A double-blind controlled trial of danazol and bromocriptine in the management of severe cyclical breast pain. Br J Clin Pract 1986;40(8):326–30.
130. Arrowsmith-Lowe T. Bromocriptine indications withdrawn. FDA Med Bull 1994;24(2).
131. Aydin Y, Atis A, Kaleli S, et al. Cabergoline versus bromocriptine for symptomatic treatment of premenstrual mastalgia: a randomised, open-label study. Eur J Obstet Gynecol Reprod Biol 2010;150(2):203–6.
132. Chan J. Magic for mastalgia with HT7. Acupuncture Med 2015;33(1):82.
133. Thicke LA, Hazelton JK, Bauer BA, et al. Acupuncture for treatment of noncyclic breast pain: a pilot study. Am J Chin Med 2011;39(06):1117–29.
134. Gregory W, Mills S, Hamed H, et al. Applied kinesiology for treatment of women with mastalgia. Breast 2001;10(1):15–9.

Lobular Neoplasia

Lilia Lunt, MD[a], Alison Coogan, MD[a], Claudia B. Perez, DO, MS[b],*

KEYWORDS

- Lobular carcinoma in situ • LCIS • Atypical lobular hyperplasia • ALH
- Pleomorphic lobular carcinoma in situ • Core needle biopsy • High-risk lesion
- Breast cancer risk

KEY POINTS

- Lobular neoplasia (LN) is a term that describes the continuum of atypical epithelial lesions originating in the terminal duct-lobular unit (TDLU) of the breast, including atypical lobular hyperplasia (ALH) and lobular carcinoma in situ (LCIS), further classified as classical LCIS (CLCIS), pleomorphic LCIS (PLCIS) and Florid LCIS (FLCIS).
- LCIS is both a risk factor and nonobligate precursor to invasive breast cancer, with an increased risk for the development of ipsilateral breast cancer and a higher incidence of invasive lobular carcinoma than the general population.
- LN leads to an increased risk of the development of breast cancer. A diagnosis of LCIS is associated with a risk of 1% to 2% a year of developing invasive carcinoma or DCIS and a 7-to-10-fold increased risk of breast cancer compared with the general population. A diagnosis of ALH is associated with a 4-to-5-fold increased risk of breast cancer compared with the general population.
- Patients diagnosed with LN should be counseled on the risk of developing invasive carcinoma and advised on current screening and chemoprevention recommendations.

INTRODUCTION

Lobular neoplasia (LN) is a term that describes the continuum of atypical epithelial lesions originating in the terminal duct-lobular unit (TDLU) of the breast.[1] To predict cancer risk, further subclassification of LN into atypical lobular hyperplasia (ALH) and lobular carcinoma in situ (LCIS) is traditionally performed. This represents a proliferation gradation from AHL to LCIS which correlates with an increase in the relative risk of the development of invasive carcinoma.[2,3] This distinction is a quantitative analysis of the degree of acini in the lobular unit filled with neoplastic cells; it is not a qualitative difference between the lesions. Therefore, it is often subjective and can be distorted by the completeness of lesion biopsy.[4]

[a] Department of Surgery, Rush University Medical Center, Rush University, 600 South Paulina Street, Chicago, IL 60612, USA; [b] Breast Surgery Oncology, Rush University Medical Center, Chicago, IL, USA
* Corresponding author. Rush University Medical Center, Rush University, Department of Surgery, 600 South Paulina Street, Chicago, IL 60612.
E-mail address: Claudia_b_perez@rush.edu

Surg Clin N Am 102 (2022) 947–963
https://doi.org/10.1016/j.suc.2022.07.001
0039-6109/22/© 2022 Elsevier Inc. All rights reserved.
surgical.theclinics.com

In 1919, Ewing first described LN as an "atypical proliferation of acinar cells" within a breast specimen.[5] Work on the disease was further advanced by Foote and Stewart in 1941.[6] They described the similarities between the cells in LCIS specimens and invasive lobular carcinoma; however, they noted that the cells in LCIS were contained by the basement membrane. Their hypothesis was that LCIS was a precursor lesion that could progress to invasive carcinoma when the atypical cells were no longer contained by the basement membrane.[6] The recommendation based on this early research was for mastectomy to prevent the development of invasive cancer.

In the 1970s, the recommendations changed when Haagensen published work demonstrating the risk of invasive cancer developing in women with LCIS was around 1% a year, significantly less than would be expected from a precursor lesion.[7] This led to the assertion that "when [LN] occurs alone without accompanying infiltrating carcinoma, it is a distinctive benign disease which predisposes to subsequent carcinoma."[7] This seminal work led to a change in the management of this lesion. Rather than a mastectomy, women began to be offered observation with close follow-up.

In modern clinical settings, LN is considered a risk factor for the development of invasive carcinoma in both breasts, and therefore, counseling focuses on surveillance and chemoprevention, rather than surgical treatments. However, a growing body of work has supported the idea that LN is a nonobligate precursor as well as a risk indicator for the development of invasive neoplasia.[8–10] This molecular research demonstrates that LN and adjacent invasive carcinoma share genetic aberrations, which supports the hypothesis that LN can transform into invasive breast cancer.[8]

PATHOLOGY

The 5th edition of the WHO classification of breast tumors divides "noninvasive lobular neoplasia" into ALH and LCIS.[1] (Lakhani) LCIS is further subdivided into classical LCIS (CLCIS), pleomorphic LCIS (PLCIS) and florid LCIS (FLCIS).[1] The differentiation between the subtypes of LCIS has gained increased importance, as current NCCN guidelines recommend surveillance or excision following percutaneous core needle biopsy (CNB) with ALH/CLCIS and excisional biopsy following PLCIS and FLCIS.[11] (Table 1).

Atypical Lobular Hyperplasia

The criteria for the diagnosis of ALH were proposed by Page and colleagues in 1985.[3] ALH is defined as a lesion for which the acini of a lobular unit are filled with small, round, or polygonal cells. To be defined as ALH rather than CLCIS, less than 50% of the acini in the affected TDLU are distended. Unlike LCIS, cellular proliferation does not occlude the lumen.[12] The difference between ALH and CLCIS is quantitative, and therefore prone to misclassification based on the completeness of the sample. Some studies have demonstrated a lack of concordance among pathologists in differentiating the 2 lesions, especially on CNB.[13]

Classic Lobular Carcinoma in Situ

The WHO definition of classic LCIS is a lesion consisting of a monomorphic population of dyshesive cells with small, uniform round nuclei and scant cytoplasm.[1] (Fig. 1) (Lakhani) The lesion is often multicentric and bilateral. To qualify as LCIS, at least half of the acini in a terminal duct lobular unit (TDLU) must be filled by neoplastic cells, which include type A and/or type B epithelial cells.[14] (Chen) Classic LCIS typically has

Table 1
Pathologic features and management recommendations for LCIS subtypes

	Classic LCIS	Pleomorphic LCIS	Florid LCIS
Pathology	May include type A or type B epithelial cells. Typically pale or eosinophilic	Nuclei are at least 4 times greater than the lymphocyte nuclei. May include multinucleation	Marked distention of the TDLU, which may include (1) little intervening stroma and/or (2) expanded acini at least one high power field
Necrosis or Calcification	Rarely present	May be present	Often present
E-Cadherin Expression	Dysfunctional	Dysfunctional	Dysfunctional
Hormone Receptor Expression	Nearly always ER/PR positive, HER2 negative	Often ER/PR positive, HER2 negative	Often ER/PR positive, HER2 negative, but more variability in expression
If diagnosed in surgical specimen	No further surgical excision No Margin assessment Increased surveillance and consideration of chemoprevention	Assess margin status and consider re-excision Increased surveillance and consideration of chemoprevention	Assess margin status and consider re-excision Increased surveillance and consideration of chemoprevention
If diagnosed on core needle biopsy	Assess pathologic and radiologic concurrence. If in agreement, no need for further surgical excision. Increased surveillance and consideration of chemoprevention	Routine surgical excision	Routine surgical excision

a strong expression of estrogen receptor and progesterone receptor, while lacking HER2 overexpression.[15] (Chen YY) Classic LCIS also usually has a loss of membrane expression of E-cadherin, an adhesion molecule, and other proteins of the cadherin–catenin complex.[16] (Dabbs) The cytoplasm is typically pale or lightly eosinophilic, as some cells contain intracytoplasmic vacuoles that may contain an eosinophilic globule. Unlike PLCIS and FLCIS, CLCIS is not associated with microcalcifications or a mass on mammography.[17] This lesion is predominantly found incidentally following tissue sampling targeting another breast abnormality.[18]

Pleomorphic Lobular Carcinoma in Situ

PLCIS was first described in 1992 by Eusebi and colleagues as a morphologic variant of LCIS.[19] PLCIS is characterized by high-grade nuclear atypia, granular eosinophilic "apocrine" cytoplasm, and prominent, central nucleoli.[1] (**Fig. 2**) PLCIS has some nuclei that are at least four times greater than the lymphocyte nucleus and/or nuclei that are equal to nuclei in high-grade ductal carcinoma in situ (DCIS).[15] Some cells may have multinucleation, although this is not required to be defined as PLCIS. Additionally, comedo necrosis and calcifications are often seen in PLCIS samples.[19] E-cadherin staining is often required to differentiate PLCIS from high-grade DCIS,

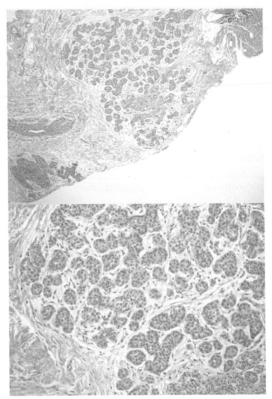

Fig. 1. Histologic features of classic lobular carcinoma in situ demonstrating the distention of the TDLU with monomorphic, dyshesive, small, round neoplastic cells with scant cytoplasm. (All figures used with permission of Dr. Indu Agarwal, Rush University Medical Center.)

as the 2 can resemble each other histologically.[16] Like classic LCIS, PLCIS lacks membrane E-cadherin. Classic LCIS is nearly always ER positive, PR positive, and HER2 negative, whereas one study found that PLCIS can be ER and PR negative in up to 48% of cases and have overexpression of HER2 in 13% of cases.[15] PLCIS can present as microcalcifications on mammography, so unlike CLCIS, PLCIS on CNB is often the targeted lesion as opposed to an incidental finding.[20]

Florid Lobular Carcinoma in Situ

FLCIS has cytologic features similar to classic LCIS but differs in that it has marked distention of the TDLU.[1] This distention of the ducts creates a confluent mass-like structure. FLCIS has at least one of the 2 architectural features: (1) little to no intervening stroma between acini and (2) minimum size of expanded acinous or duct filling of at least one high power field (an area equivalent of approximately 40–50 cells in diameter).[21] (**Fig. 3**) This lesion can often present with comedo necrosis and calcifications, but these features are not required for diagnosis.[1] FLCIS diagnosed on CNB also often represents the targeted lesion. FLCIS with necrosis often presents with calcifications and FLCIS without necrosis can seem as a nonmass enhancement on mammography.[22]

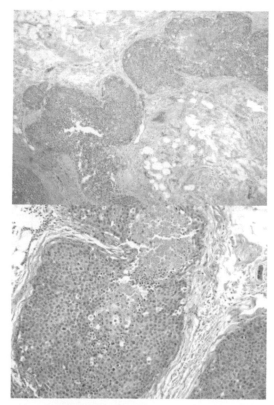

Fig. 2. Histologic features of pleomorphic lobular carcinoma in situ demonstrating the TDLU distended by large dyshesive cells with abundant cytoplasm and nuclei with pronounced atypia and pleomorphism. (All figures used with permission of Dr. Indu Agarwal, Rush University Medical Center.)

GENETICS

Classical LN typically has phenotypical characteristics consistent with the luminal A molecular subtype of less aggressive ER-positive breast cancers. These lesions are characterized by strong ER and PR expression, lack of expression of HER2 and p53, low proliferation (as defined by Ki-67), and low grade.[23]

E-Cadherin is a cell adhesion protein expressed in epithelial cells encoded by the CDH1 gene. The protein complexes with beta-, gamma-, alpha- and p120-catenin subtypes on the cell membrane. The alteration of the E-cadherin adhesion complex is a defining characteristic of LN and invasive lobular carcinoma.[24,25] Lack of significant downregulation of E-cadherin expression is observed in 95% of ALH, LCIS, and ILC lesions.[26] When LN lesions are evaluated by immunohistochemistry, they are negative for E-cadherin and p120-catenin is localized to the cytoplasm, rather than the membrane. This indicates that the alteration of the E-cadherin adhesion complex is an early step occurring in the hyperplasia phase before progression to invasive disease. However, studies have demonstrated that changes in the CDH1 gene locus, most commonly losses of 16q, occur in LCIS and ILC, but not ALH.[24,27]

Traditionally, LCIS has been considered a risk factor for the development of invasive carcinoma and managed accordingly. However, studies have previously demonstrated that synchronous LN and ILC may be clonally related, and both arise from a

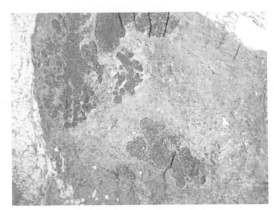

Fig. 3. Histologic features of florid lobular carcinoma in situ demonstrating the marked distention of the TDLU including little intervening stroma. (All figures used with permission of Dr. Indu Agarwal, Rush University Medical Center.)

common ancestral lesion.[9,10,28,29] Recent work by Lee and colleagues examined the clonal relatedness of LCIS and synchronously diagnosed DCIS and ILC and demonstrated that LCIS is clonally related and can progress to DCIS/ILC.[8] Additionally, the LCIS that was closely related to more advanced lesions had a higher level of intralesional genetic heterogeneity, specifically those lesions with an APOBEC mutation (a mutation associated with genetic instability).[30] The authors hypothesized that the increase in mutagenesis associated with the upregulation of APOBEC3B can promote progression of LCIS to ILC.[8]

BREAST CANCER RISK

Lobular neoplasia has traditionally been considered a risk factor for the development of breast cancer, as opposed to a precursor lesion like DCIS, based on early work demonstrating that women with the lesion had a risk of both ductal and lobular subtypes of invasive cancer in bilateral breasts.[3,31,32] However, recent work has demonstrated that women with an LCIS diagnosis have an increased risk of carcinoma in the ipsilateral breast, and a higher risk of developing ILC.[9,32,33] A recent study of the Mayo Benign Breast Disease Cohort demonstrated that following a diagnosis of ALH, patients have a 2:1 predominance of ipsilateral compared with contralateral breast cancer that was most marked in the first 5 years after atypia diagnosis.[34] Additionally, genetic analysis of adjacent LN and invasive cancer has demonstrated that genetic alterations found in the invasive tumor are often present in the LN lesion.[35] This, coupled with the molecular work demonstrating the relationship between clonal groups in LCIS and synchronous ILC/DCIS supports the hypothesis that LCIS is both a risk factor and nonobligate precursor to invasive breast cancer.

Recent and historic case series demonstrate a 7-to-10-fold increase in the risk of breast cancer development after a diagnosis of LCIS and a 4-to-5-fold increase after a diagnosis of ALH.[3,33,36–38] As previously discussed, the difference between these 2 lesions is subjective and can be altered by the completeness of the biopsy and differences in pathology review. In studies with long-term follow-up, an 11% to 28% 15-year risk of developing either DCIS or invasive cancer has been reported for patients with LN.[37,38] Collins and colleagues recently reviewed all pathology reports within the Partners Health care System from 1987 to 2010 and stratified BC risk (DCIS or IC) based on pathology. They reported a 10-year risk of 21% and 24% for ALH and LCIS, respectively.[39] In a longitudinal single-institution study, investigators at Memorial Sloane Kettering Cancer Center (MSKCC) demonstrated a 2% annual incidence of breast cancer in women with LCIS.[36] Interestingly, this study reported that this risk was not impacted by patient age or family history of breast cancer. However, one factor that has been demonstrated to impact risk is the extent of LN found in a breast sample.[39] A recently published study of 2 independent cohorts demonstrated that the risk of development of breast cancer increased significantly as the number of foci of ALH increased.[40] They reported an RR of 2.58, 3.49 and 4.97 for 1, 2, greater than 3 foci of ALH ($P = .001$).[40] It is important to note that traditional models for predicting breast cancer risk are not accurate in women with LN. The Tyrer-Cuzick model and Breast Cancer Risk Assessment Tool (Gail Model) are both inaccurate at predicting future outcomes in patients with LN and tend to overpredict risk.[41,42]

CLINICAL MANAGEMENT

The role of the surgeon in the diagnosis and treatment of LN is to determine pathologic and mammographic concordance and to recommend an appropriate strategy for long-term breast cancer risk reduction. LCIS is a relatively uncommon breast lesion, present in 0.5% to 4% of benign breast biopsies.[43,44] However, the incidence of identification is increasing. In a study of the Surveillance, Epidemiology and End Results (SEER) database, the rate of LCIS detection from 2000 to 2009 increased from 2 to 2.75 per 100,000, demonstrating a 38% increase.[45] This increased incidence can partially be explained by increasing rates of mammography and CNB for screening abnormalities. LN is most frequently identified as an incidental finding on CNB performed for other reasons.[18] Therefore, as mammogram rates and resolution increase, the number of CNBs performed and rate of LN diagnosed is increasing.

CORE NEEDLE BIOPSY AND SURGICAL EXCISION

The current National Comprehensive Cancer Network (NCCN) guidelines recommend that when LN is diagnosed on a CNB, the patient may proceed with either screening or surgical excisional biopsy of the lesion.[11] More specifically, screening includes physical examination, and mammogram ± ultrasound at 6 months following CNB to assess for stability of the lesion.[11] The ASBrS Society supports these recommendations, stating that if LN is found on CNB, the surgeon may decide to either excise the lesion or observe with clinical follow-up including examination and imaging, unless: the biopsy results are discordant with imaging, there was limited sampling of the lesion, or another high-risk lesion was identified on biopsy.[46] (ASBrS) This recent change in guidelines reflects a large number of contemporary, high-quality studies demonstrating an acceptably low risk of invasive carcinoma identified on excisional biopsy following a diagnosis of ALH or classic LCIS on CNB.[47–65] These studies demonstrate a low risk of upstaging when pathologic and imaging findings are concordant (and classic LCIS is the highest risk finding on CNB.) (**Table 2**) If surgical excision is performed, current practices treat CLCIS as a high-risk lesion and therefore it is not necessary to access margin status.[11] The goal of the biopsy is diagnostic; in other words, to investigate for adjacent DCIS or invasive carcinoma, not perform a complete excision of the lesion.

PLCIS and FLCIS are morphologic subtypes of LCIS described in the 5th edition of the World Health Organization Classification of Tumors of the Breast that have genomic alterations associated with more aggressive breast cancer and are more frequently associated with invasive carcinoma and DCIS.[22,66] Kuba and colleagues

Table 2
Upgrade rates for individual studies, reported as rates of imaging-concordant classic lobular neoplasia assessed by either surgical excision or clinical/imaging follow-up

The Rate of Upgrade of Lobular Neoplasia on Excisional Biopsy

Study	Years	# of Biopsies	Upgrade Rate					
			LN		ALH		LCIS	
Hwang et al,[47] 2008	1996–2006	221	1%	(2/221)	NR		NR	
Menon et al,[48] 2008	1998–2010	44	11%	(5/44)	NR		NR	
Purdie et al,[49] 2010	2000–2009	45	16%	(7/45)	NR		NR	
Niell et al,[50] 2012	2005–2010	47	9%	(4/47)	6%	(1/16)	10%	(3/31)
Rendi et al,[51] 2012	2003–2009	67	4%	(3/67)	2%	(1/47)	5%	(1/20)
Shah-Khan et al,[52] 2012	1993–2010	166	1%	(2/166)	1%	(1/124)	3%	(1/32)
Atkins et al,[53] 2013	2000–2010	43	0%	(0/43)	NR		NR	
Chaudhary et al,[54] 2013	2006–2011	87	3%	(3/87)	0%	(0/22)	5%	(3/65)
Murray et al,[55] 2013	2004–2009	72	3%	(2/72)	7%	(2/30)	0%	(0/40)
Mooney et al,[56] 2016	2003–2014	74	14%	(10/74)	7%	(3/43)	23%	(7/31)
Nakhlis et al,[57] 2016	2004–2014	77	3%	(2/77)	0%	(0/49)	12%	(2/17)
Sen et al,[58] 2016	2006–2013	442	4%	(17/442)	8%	(9/107)	2%	(8/335)
Susnik et al,[59] 2016	2008–2012	228	4%	(8/228)	3%	(6/182)	4%	(2/46)
Muller et al,[60] 2018	2000–2016	87	3%	(3/87)	3%	(3/87)	NA	
Schmidt et al,[61] 2018	2001–2014	115	4%	(5/115)	NR		NR	
Holbrook et al,[62] 2019	2005–2012	55	0%	(0/55)	NR		NR	
Li et al,[63] 2020	2015–2019	31	0%	(0/31)	0%	(0/19)	0%	(0/12)
Pride et al,[64] 2021	2008–2019	78	14%	(11/78)	NR		14%	(11/78)
Laws et al,[65] 2022	2015–2019	97	0%	(0/97)	0%	(0/72)	0%	(0/25)

Abbreviations: ALH, atypical lobular hyperplasia; LCIS, lobular carcinoma in situ; LN, lobular neoplasia.

recently performed a retrospective review of FLCIS and PLCIS diagnosed on CNB and found an upgrade rate of 25% for PLCIS and 17% for FLCIS.[67] This supports the previous literature demonstrating a significantly higher upgrade rate on surgical excision of nonclassic LCIS compared with CLCIS, with upgrade rates ranging from 25% to 60%, supporting routine surgical excision.[68–71] Following excisional biopsy for PLCIS, positive margins are often present as PLCIS can be a diffuse and extensive lesion. This is an area of study without a clear consensus. A recent survey of American breast surgeons revealed that when confronted with PLCIS at surgical margins, 53% recommended no re-excision, 24% always re-excised, and 23% sometimes re-excised.[72] An additional higher risk group is patients with multifocal LN, defined as greater than 4 terminal ductal units on CN. This group has an increased risk of invasive carcinoma on excision.[40]

SURGICAL GUIDELINES

For patients undergoing excisional biopsy for LN, there is no need to assess margin status for specimens for which the highest risk lesion is classic LCIS. Additionally, for patients undergoing a lumpectomy for DCIS or IC, the presence of CLCIS within the specimen or at the margin does not change surgical management.[3] Studies have demonstrated that the presence of LCIS within a specimen following breast conservation therapy does not increase local recurrence.[37,69,73] If LN is found in a breast specimen following reduction mammoplasty, the recommendation is similar to those found on CNB, including surveillance and consideration of chemoprevention.

As discussed above, there is little high-quality evidence on the management of positive margins for PLCIS and FLCIS. Based on survey evidence, around 50% of breast surgeons re-excise or consider re-excision when PLCIS is found at the margin of a specimen.[72] Small, retrospective studies show a recurrence rate ranging from 0% to 57%.[68–71] Khoury and colleagues published a multi-institution study demonstrating a recurrent rate of 19.4% in 31 patients with pure PLCIS following excisional biopsy. 4 of the 6 recurrences had positive margins on initial biopsy.[74] Downs-Kelly and colleagues published a report of 20 patients with pure PLCIS on excisional biopsy in which 5 patients had a positive margin following excision and 1 of those positive margin patients recurred. In this study, no patients with a negative margin developed invasive cancer, DCIS, or PLCIS at the excision site.[69]

RISK REDUCTION STRATEGIES
Surveillance

There are 3 societies that set the radiographic screening guidelines for breast cancer: the NCCN, the American College of Radiology, and the American Cancer Society. All 3 of these organizations recommend annual screening mammography for patients diagnosed with LCIS or ALH along with a breast exam performed by a health care provider every 6 to 12 months.[11,75,76] The society guidelines give recommendations for women specifically with LCIS and women who have a calculated greater than 20% lifetime risk of developing BC. This group is composed of women with gene mutations and those who have a calculated risk by breast cancer risk models. As previously discussed, these model systems have a poor predictive power in women with LN.[41,42] The risk based on studies with greater than 15-year follow-up seems to be around 2% each year for LCIS and 1% each year for ALH.[36] Therefore, for women with an LCIS diagnosis, the lifetime risk of developing breast cancer can exceed 20% based on age at diagnosis.

The recommendations for breast MRI are currently under debate with variations between organizations. The NCCN recommends the consideration of an annual breast MRI for women with LCIS or ALH.[11] The American College of Radiology recommends an annual MRI for women with greater than 20% lifetime risk of breast cancer and recommends considering MRI for women with 15% to 20% lifetime risk.[75] The guidelines define risk from LCIS to be between 10% and 20% and therefore recommend the consideration of MRI, especially if other risk factors are present or if the patient has dense breast tissue.[75] A retrospective study by Nadler and colleagues specifically looked at a group of women with high-risk lesions including LN and extremely dense breasts.[77] They demonstrated that cancer detection rate (CDR) and false positive (FP) rate were 6.1% and 21%, which is comparable to previous work published for BRCA carriers. Additionally, they determined that the population of patients with LN that benefited the most from additional screening was women with a family history of BC and not on antiestrogen therapy.[77] Currently, the ACS recommends only considering annual MRI for women with LN.[76] This is based on the difference in cancer characteristics between women with LCIS and women whose risk is due to BRCA mutations or strong family history. A recent large cohort study at MSKCC demonstrated in 776 women with LCIS that adjuvant MRI screening in the first 3 years following diagnosis did not translate to increased CDR or earlier stage of diagnosis.[78] Additionally, women who received MRI screening had significantly more benign biopsies compared with the control group (36% vs 13%, $P<.0001$). The authors argue that unlike the young high-risk mutation carriers, who frequently develop high-grade invasive cancer in the interval between annual mammogram screening, patients with LCIS typically develop low-grade, ER + cancers that are detected at an early stage regardless of the type of screening protocol used.[78,79]

Chemoprevention

In 1998, the results of the National Surgical Adjuvant Breast and Bowel Projected (NSABP) Breast Cancer Prevention Trial (BCPT P-1) were published demonstrating the effectiveness of tamoxifen for breast cancer prevention.[80] In this landmark study, women with LCIS comprised 6.2% of the 13,338 participants and the risk of the development of breast cancer was reduced by more than 50%.[80] The NSABP Study of Tamoxifen and Raloxifene (STAR P-2) trial further confirmed these results for raloxifene with 19,747 patients (9.2% with LCIS).[81] Following the results of the SERM trials, the Map.3 trial studied the effect of exemestane in the prevention of breast cancer in high-risk postmenopausal women and found a 65% risk reduction.[82] This population included women with ALH and LCIS diagnosis. In the subgroup analysis of the Breast Cancer Prevention Trial comparing tamoxifen versus placebo, a risk reduction of 86% and 56% was seen for women with AH and LCIS, respectively.[80] Additionally, the IBIS-II trial subset analysis of women with AH and LCIS demonstrates a 69% risk reduction for women receiving anastrozole versus placebo.[83] All of these positive findings have led many organizations including the NCCN and ACS recommend chemoprevention with SERMs or aromatase inhibitors for women with LN.[11,76]

Despite these extremely encouraging findings, the rates of women with LN currently using chemoprevention are very low, between 20% and 30%.[84–86] Tamoxifen therapy can increase menopausal symptoms including sexual and gynecologic disturbances, leading to decreased quality of life. Additionally, the side effects of thromboembolic events and endometrial cancer may discourage patients from starting chemoprevention. In studies, the most cited reasons given by patients for declining chemoprevention were fear of endometrial cancer, thromboembolic disease, and menopause symptoms.[87,88] A recent proof of the principle study performed at MD Anderson Cancer Center looked at using a system-level performance improvement program to target prevention therapy uptake. They audited eligible patients with a diagnosis of AH/LCIS and provided clinical performance feedback to providers based on the prescription of chemoprevention. Following the initiative, adherence among patients was 78% for those with a new diagnosis and 48% for those with an existing diagnosis.[89]

A recent multicenter randomized trial looking at a 5 mg/d of Tamoxifen administered for 3 years in hormone-sensitive breast intraepithelial neoplasia (including ADH, LCIS, and DCIS) demonstrated a similar result to the 20 mg/d for 5-year dosing in the original studies.[90] The lower dose produced no increase in adverse events compared with placebo. Additionally, when assessing for quality of life and adherence, the only significant finding was a 1.5-fold higher incidence of hot flashes in the Tamoxifen versus placebo group.[90] (DeCensi) Unlike the full dose studies, adherence was the same in both study arms.[80–82,90]

Risk-Reducing Surgery

In the modern era of breast surgery, mastectomy for the treatment of LN is rarely used as a treatment option.[91] Standard treatment for this lesion includes lifelong surveillance and medical risk reduction. Based on the evidence that LN increases the risk of the development of DCIS and invasive carcinoma in both breasts, historically, the surgical treatment recommended was bilateral prophylactic mastectomy without lymph node assessment for risk reduction. The NCCN guidelines support this approach, but emphasize that while BPM can be considered, risk-reducing medical therapy is the preferred approach.[11] Based on a recent longitudinal study performed at MSKCC, 5% of women with LCIS pursue a BPM for risk reduction.[36] While BPM does not eliminate the chance of breast cancer development entirely, a contemporary case-cohort study demonstrates a 95% risk reduction in a large community practice setting.[92] Nipple-sparing mastectomies are becoming more common due to improved cosmetic results and a growing body of evidence suggests that this procedure is oncologically safe.[93,94] A recent study of the National Cancer Database (NCDB) looked at surgical treatment following an LCIS diagnosis whereby 84.8% received surgical excision, 5.4% received no surgery, 5.1% received bilateral mastectomy and 4% received unilateral mastectomy. The results demonstrate that nearly as many patients received the appropriate risk reduction surgery as the inappropriate option, which is a concern.[91]

Women considering risk-reducing surgery should be carefully counseled on the possible effects of surgery on body image and sexual functioning. Additionally, if the patient desires reconstruction, a plastic surgery consultation should be provided so that the patient can gain an understanding of the expected cosmetic result. Overall, the decision to undergo prophylactic bilateral mastectomy for LN should include a thorough discussion of the risks and benefits including the medical risk reduction options available and the effect of surgery on quality of life.[95] While not the first recommended treatment option, it may be reasonable for women with additional risk factors and/or challenging mammographic surveillance.

CLINICS CARE POINTS

- Following an LN diagnosis, women should receive a screening mammogram annually and a clinical breast examination every 6 to 12 months. The use of MRI for screening in patients with LN is currently debated: the National Comprehensive Cancer Network, the American College of Radiology, and the American Cancer Society all recommend considering annual MRI for patients with LN, but recent studies have not demonstrated an improvement in cancer detection rate (CDR) or earlier stage of diagnosis.

- The current NCCN and ASBrS guidelines recommend that when classic LCIS or ALH is diagnosed on a core needle biopsy (CNB), the patient may proceed with either screening (consisting of a mammogram and clinical examination at 6 months) or excisional biopsy of the lesion. Based on high upstage rates of invasive carcinoma/DCIS, PLCIS and FLCIS lesions should be surgically excised if found on CNB.

- For patients undergoing excisional biopsy for LN, there is no need to assess margin status for specimens for which the highest risk lesion is classic LCIS. Studies have demonstrated that the presence of LCIS within a specimen following breast conservation therapy does not increase local recurrence.

- The NCCN and ACS recommend chemoprevention with SERMs or aromatase inhibitors for women with LN based on many RCTs that have demonstrated a greater than 50% reduction in the risk of developing invasive cancer.

DISCLOSURE

The authors have nothing to disclose.

REFERENCES

1. Lakhani SR, International Agency for Research on Cancer. 2nd edition. WHO classification of breast tumours: WHO classification of tumours, vol. 2. Lyon, France: IARC; 2019. Who Classification of Tumours Editorial Board.
2. London SJ, Connolly JL, Schnitt SJ, et al. A prospective study of benign breast disease and the risk of breast cancer. JAMA 1992;267:941–4.
3. Page DL, Dupont WD, Rogers LW, et al. Atypical hyperplastic lesions of the female breast: a long-term follow-up study. Cancer 1985;55:2698–708.
4. Simpson PT, Gale T, Fulford LG, et al. The diagnosis and management of pre-invasive breast disease: pathology of atypical lobular hyperplasia and lobular carcinoma in situ. Breast Cancer Res 2003;5(5):258–62.
5. Ewing J. Neoplastic diseases: a textbook on tumors. Philadelphia: WB Saunders; 1919.
6. Foote FW Jr, Stewart FW. Lobular carcinoma *in situ*. A rare form of mammary cancer. Am J Pathol 1941;17:491–6.
7. Haagensen CD, Lane N, Lattes R, et al. Lobular neoplasia (so-called lobular carcinoma *in situ*) of the breast. Cancer 1978;42:737–69.
8. Lee JY, Schizas M, Geyer FC, et al. Lobular Carcinomas *In Situ* Display Intralesion Genetic Heterogeneity and Clonal Evolution in the Progression to Invasive Lobular Carcinoma. Clin Cancer Res 2019;25(2):674–86.
9. Andrade VP, Ostrovnaya I, Seshan VE, et al. Clonal relatedness between lobular carcinoma in situ and synchronous malignant lesions. Breast Cancer Res 2012; 14(4):R103.
10. Begg CB, Ostrovnaya I, Carniello JV, et al. Clonal relationships between lobular carcinoma in situ and other breast malignancies. Breast Cancer Res 2016;18:66.
11. National Comprehensive Cancer Network. Breast Cancer Screening and Diagnosis. Available at: https://www.nccn.org/professionals/physician_gls/pdf/breast-screening.pdf. Accessed April 1, 2022.
12. Page DL, Rogers LW. Combined histologic and cytologic criteria for the diagnosis of mammary atypical ductal hyperplasia. Hum Pathol 1992;23(10):1095–7.
13. Jain RK, Mehta R, Dimitrov R, et al. Atypical ductal hyperplasia: interobserver and intraobserver variability. Mod Pathol 2011;24:917–23.
14. Chen YYDT, King TA, Palacios J, et al. Lobular carcinoma in situ. In: Board TWCE, editor. Breast Tumours. Lyon (France): International Agency for Research on Cancer; 2019. p. 71–4.
15. Chen YY, Hwang ES, Roy R, et al. Genetic and phenotypic characteristics of pleomorphic lobular carcinoma in situ of the breast. Am J Surg Pathol 2009;33(11): 1683–94.
16. Dabbs DJ, Schnitt SJ, Geyer FC, et al. Lobular neoplasia of the breast revisited with emphasis on the role of E-cadherin immunohistochemistry. Am J Surg Pathol 2013;37(7):1–11.
17. Beute BJ, Kalisher L, Hutter RV. Lobular carcinoma in situ of the breast: clinical, pathologic, and mammographic features. AJR Am J Roentgenol 1991;157(2): 257–65.
18. Maxwell AJ, Clements K, Dodwell DJ, et al. The radiological features, diagnosis and management of screen-detected lobular neoplasia of the breast: Findings from the Sloane Project. Breast 2016;27:109–15.
19. Eusebi V, Magalhaes F, Azzopardi JG. Pleomorphic lobular carcinoma of the breast: an aggressive tumor showing apocrine differentiation. Hum Pathol 1992;23(6):655–62.

20. Sneige N, Wang J, Baker BA, et al. Clinical, histopathologic, and biologic features of pleomorphic lobular (ductal-lobular) carcinoma in situ of the breast: a report of 24 cases. Mod Pathol 2002;15(10):1044–50.

21. Alvarado-Cabrero I, Picon Coronel G, Valencia Cedillo R, et al. Florid lobular intra-epithelial neoplasia with signet ring cells, central necrosis and calcifications: a clinicopathological and immunohistochemical analysis of ten cases associated with invasive lobular carcinoma. Arch Med Res 2010;41(6):436–41.

22. Shamir ER, Chen YY, Chu T, et al. Pleomorphic and florid lobular carcinoma in situ variants of the breast: a clinicopathologic study of 85 cases with and without inva-sive carcinoma from a single academic center. Am J Surg Pathol 2019;43: 399–408.

23. Lopez-Garcia MA, Geyer FC, Lacroix-Triki M, et al. Breast cancer precursors re-visited: molecular features and progression pathways. Histopathology 2010;57: 171–92.

24. Mastracci T, Tjan S, Bane A, et al. E-cadherin alterations in atypical lobular hyper-plasia and lobular carcinoma in situ of the breast. Mod Pathol 2005;18:741–51.

25. Sarrio D, Moreno-Bueno G, Hardisson D, et al. Epigenetic and genetic alterations of APC and CDH1 genes in lobular breast cancer: Relationships with abnormal E-cadherin and catenin expression and microsatellite instability. Int J Cancer 2003;106:208–15.

26. Derksen PW, Liu X, Saridin F, et al. Somatic inactivation of E-cadherin and p53 in mice leads to metastatic lobular mammary carcinoma through induction of anoi-kis resistance and angiogenesis. Cancer Cell 2006;10:437–49.

27. Weigelt B, Geyer FC, Natrajan R, et al. The molecular underpinning of lobular his-tological growth pattern: a genome-wide transcriptomic analysis of invasive lobular carcinomas and grade- and molecular subtype-matched invasive ductal carcinomas of no special type. J Pathol 2010;220:45–57.

28. Lu YJ, Osin P, Lakhani SR, et al. Comparative genomic hybridization analysis of lobular carcinoma in situ and atypical lobular hyperplasia and potential roles for gains and losses of genetic material in breast neoplasia. Cancer Res 1998;58: 4721–7.

29. Ciriello G, Gatza ML, Beck AH, et al. Comprehensive molecular portraits of inva-sive lobular breast cancer. Cell 2015;163:506–19.

30. Swanton C, McGranahan N, Starrett GJ, et al. APOBEC enzymes: mutagenic fuel for cancer evolution and heterogeneity. Cancer Discov 2015;5:704–12.

31. Li CI, Malone KE, Saltzman BS, et al. Risk of invasive breast carcinoma among women diagnosed with ductal carcinoma in situ and lobular carcinoma in situ, 1988–2001. Cancer 2006;106(10):2104–12.

32. Reis-Filho JS, Pusztai L. Gene expression profiling in breast cancer: classifica-tion, prognostication, and prediction. Lancet 2011;378(9805):1812–23.

33. Dupont WD, Page DL. Risk factors for breast cancer in women with proliferative breast disease. N Engl J Med 1985;312(3):146–51.

34. Hartmann LC, Schaid DJ, Woods JE, et al. Efficacy of bilateral prophylactic mas-tectomy in women with a family history of breast cancer. N Engl J Med 1999; 340(2):77–84.

35. Page DL, Kidd TE Jr, Dupont WD, et al. Lobular neoplasia of the breast: higher risk for subsequent invasive cancer predicted by more extensive disease. Hum Pathol 1991;22:1232–9.

36. King TA, Pilewskie M, Muhsen S, et al. Lobular Carcinoma in Situ: A 29-Year Lon-gitudinal Experience Evaluating Clinicopathologic Features and Breast Cancer Risk. J Clin Oncol 2015;33(33):3945–52.

37. Bodian CA, Perzin KH, Lattes R. Lobular neoplasia. Long term risk of breast cancer and relation to other factors. Cancer 1996;78(5):1024–34.
38. Chuba PJ, Hamre MR, Yap J, et al. Bilateral risk for subsequent breast cancer after lobular carcinoma-in-situ: Analysis of Surveillance, Epidemiology, and End Results data. J Clin Oncol 2005;23:5534–41.
39. Collins LC, Aroner SA, Connolly JL, et al. Breast cancer risk by extent and type of atypical hyperplasia: An update from the Nurses' Health Studies. Cancer 2016; 122(4):515–20.
40. Degnim AC, Dupont WD, Radisky DC, et al. Extent of atypical hyperplasia stratifies breast cancer risk in 2 independent cohorts of women. Cancer 2016; 122(19):2971–8.
41. Valero MG, Zabor EC, Park A, et al. The Tyrer-Cuzick Model Inaccurately Predicts Invasive Breast Cancer Risk in Women With LCIS. Ann Surg Oncol 2020;27(3): 736–40.
42. Pankratz VS, Hartmann LC, Degnim AC, et al. Assessment of the accuracy of the Gail model in women with atypical hyperplasia. J Clin Oncol 2008;26(33):5374–9.
43. Frykberg ER. Lobular carcinoma in situ of the breast. Breast J 1999;5:296–303.
44. Hussain M, Cunnick GH. Management of lobular carcinoma in-situ and atypical lobular hyperplasia of the breast: A review. Eur J Surg Oncol 2011;37:279–89.
45. Portschy PR, Marmor S, Nzara R, et al. Trends in incidence and management of lobular carcinoma in situ: A population-based analysis. Ann Surg Oncol 2013;20: 3240–6.
46. The American Society of Breast Surgeons. Position Statement on Screening Mammography. Available at: https://www.breastsurgeons.org/docs/statements/ Position-Statement-on-Screening-Mammography.pdf. Assessed April 1, 2022.
47. Hwang H, Barke LD, Mendelson EB, et al. Atypical lobular hyperplasia and classic lobular carcinoma in situ in core biopsy specimens: routine excision is not necessary. Mod Pathol 2008;21:1208–16.
48. Menon S, Porter GJ, Evans AJ, et al. The significance of lobular neoplasia on needle core biopsy of the breast. Virch Arch 2008;452:473–9.
49. Purdie CA, McLean D, Stormonth E, et al. Management of in situ lobular neoplasia detected on needle core biopsy of breast. J Clin Pathol 2010;63: 987–93.
50. Niell B, Specht M, Gerade B, et al. Is excisional biopsy required after a breast core biopsy yields lobular neoplasia? AJR Am J Roentgenol 2012;199:929–35.
51. Rendi MH, Dintzis SM, Lehman CD, et al. Lobular in-situ neoplasia on breast core needle biopsy: imaging indication and pathologic extent can identify which patients require excisional biopsy. Ann Surg Oncol 2012;19:914–21.
52. Shah-Khan MG, Geiger XJ, Reynolds C, et al. Long-term follow-up of lobular neoplasia (atypical lobular hyperplasia/lobular carcinoma in situ) diagnosed on core needle biopsy. Ann Surg Oncol 2012;19:3131–8.
53. Atkins KA, Cohen MA, Nicholson B, et al. Atypical lobular hyperplasia and lobular carcinoma in situ at core breast biopsy: use of careful radiologic-pathologic correlation to recommend excision or observation. Radiology 2013;269:340–7.
54. Chaudhary S, Lawrence L, McGinty G, et al. Classic lobular neoplasia on core biopsy: a clinical and radio-pathologic correlation study with follow-up excision biopsy. Mod Pathol 2013;26:762–71.
55. Murray MP, Luedtke C, Liberman L, et al. Classic lobular carcinoma in situ and atypical lobular hy- perplasia at percutaneous breast core biopsy: outcomes of prospective excision. Cancer 2013;119:1073–9.

56. Mooney KL, Bassett LW, Apple SK. Upgrade rates of high-risk breast lesions diagnosed on core needle biopsy: a single-institution experience and literature review. Mod Pathol 2016;29(12):1471–84.

57. Nakhlis F, Gilmore L, Gelman R, et al. Incidence of adjacent synchronous invasive carcinoma and/or ductal carcinoma in-situ in patients with lobular neoplasia on core biopsy: results from a prospective multi-institutional registry (TBCRC 020). Ann Surg Oncol 2016;23:722–8.

58. Sen LQ, Berg WA, Hooley RJ, et al. Core breast biopsies showing lobular carcinoma in situ should be excised and surveillance is reasonable for atypical lobular hyperplasia. AJR Am J Roentgenol 2016;207:1132–45.

59. Susnik B, Day D, Abeln E, et al. Surgical outcomes of lobular neoplasia diagnosed in core biopsy: prospective study of 316 cases. Clin Breast Cancer 2016;16:507–13.

60. Muller KE, Roberts E, Zhao L, et al. Isolated atypical lobular hyperplasia diagnosed on breast biopsy: low upgrade rate on subse- quent excision with long-term follow-up. Arch Pathol Lab Med 2018;142:391–5.

61. Schmidt H, Arditi B, Wooster M, et al. Observation versus excision of lobular neoplasia on core needle biopsy of the breast. Breast Cancer Res Treat 2018; 168(3):649–54.

62. Holbrook AI, Hanley K, Jeffers C, et al. Triaging Atypical Lobular Hyperplasia and Lobular Carcinoma In Situ on Percutaneous Core Biopsy to Surgery or Observation: Assiduous Radiologic-Pathologic Correlation Works, Quantitating Extent of Disease Does Not. Arch Pathol Lab Med 2019;143(5):621–7.

63. Li X, Ma Z, Styblo TM, Arciero CA, Wang H, Cohen MA. Management of high-risk breast lesions diagnosed on core biopsies and experiences from prospective high risk breast lesion conferences at an academic institution. Breast cancer research and. treatment 2021;185(3):573–81.

64. Pride RM, Jimenez RE, Hoskin TL, et al. Upgrade at excisional biopsy after a core needle biopsy diagnosis of classic lobular carcinoma in situ. Surgery 2021; 169(3):644–8.

65. Laws A, Katlin F, Nakhlis F, et al. Atypical Lobular Hyperplasia and Classic Lobular Carcinoma In Situ Can Be Safely Managed Without Surgical Excision. Ann Surg Oncol 2022;29(3):1660–7.

66. Nakhlis F, Harrison BT, Giess CS, et al. Evaluating the rate of upgrade to invasive breast cancer and/or ductal carcinoma in situ following a core biopsy diagnosis of non-classic lobular carcinoma in situ. Ann Surg Oncol 2019;26:55–61.

67. Kuba MG, Murray MP, Coffey K, et al. Morphologic subtypes of lobular carcinoma in situ diagnosed on core needle biopsy: clinicopathologic features and findings at follow-up excision. Mod Pathol 2021;34(8):1495–506.

68. Flanagan MR, Rendi MH, Calhoun KE, et al. Pleomorphic lobular carcinoma in situ: radiologic-pathologic features and clinical management. Ann Surg Oncol 2015;22:4263–9.

69. Downs-Kelly E, Bell D, Perkins GH, et al. Clinical implications of margin involvement by pleomorphic lobular carcinoma in situ. Arch Pathol Lab Med 2011;135:737–43.

70. Sullivan ME, Khan SA, Sullu Y, et al. Lobular carcinoma in situ variants in breast cores: potential for misdiagnosis, upgrade rates at surgical excision, and practical implications. Arch Pathol Lab Med 2010;134:1024–8.

71. Chivukula M, Haynik DM, Brufsky A, et al. Pleomorphic lobular carcinoma in situ (PLCIS) on breast core needle biopsies: clinical significance and immunoprofile. Am J Surg Pathol 2008;32(11):1721–6.

72. Blair SL, Emerson DK, Kulkarni S, et al. Breast surgeon's survey: no consensus for surgical treatment of pleomorphic lobular carcinoma in situ. Breast J 2013; 19(1):116–8.
73. Moran M, Haffty BG. Lobular carcinoma in situ as a component of breast cancer: the long-term outcome in patients treated with breast conservation therapy. Int J Radiat Oncol Biol Phys 1998;40(2):353–8.
74. Khoury T, Karabakhtsian RG, Mattson D, et al. Pleomorphic lobular carcinoma in situ of the breast: clinicopathological review of 47 cases. Histopathology 2014;64:981–93.
75. Monticciolo DL, Newell MS, Moy L, et al. Breast Cancer Screening in Women at Higher-Than-Average Risk: Recommendations From the ACR. J Am Coll Radiol 2018;15(3 Pt A):408–14.
76. American Cancer Society. Lobular Carcinoma in Situ. Available at: https://www.cancer.org/cancer/breast-cancer/non-cancerous-breast-conditions/lobular-carcinoma-in-situ.html. Accessed April 1, 2022.
77. Nadler M, Al-Attar H, Warner E, et al. MRI surveillance for women with dense breasts and a previous breast cancer and/or high risk lesion. Breast 2017;34:77–82.
78. King TA, Muhsen S, Patil S, et al. Is there a role for routine screening MRI in women with LCIS? Breast Cancer Res Treat 2013;142(2):445–53.
79. Tilanus-Linthorst MM, Obdeijn IM, Hop WC, et al. BRCA1 mutation and young age predict fast breast cancer growth in the Dutch, United Kingdom, and Canadian magnetic resonance imaging screening trials. Clin Cancer Res 2007;13:7357–62.
80. Fisher B, Costantino JP, Wickerham DL, et al. Tamoxifen for prevention of breast cancer: report of the National Surgical Adjuvant Breast and Bowel Project P-1 Study. J Natl Cancer Inst 1998;90(18):1371–88.
81. Vogel VG, Costantino JP, Wickerham DL, et al. Effects of tamoxifen vs raloxifene on the risk of developing invasive breast cancer and other disease outcomes: the NSABP Study of Tamoxifen and Raloxifene (STAR) P-2 trial. JAMA 2006;295(23):2727–41.
82. Goss PE, Ingle JN, Ales-Martinez JE, et al. Exemestane for breast-cancer prevention in postmenopausal women. N Engl J Med 2011;364(25):2381–91.
83. Cuzick J, Sestak I, Forbes JF, et al. IBIS-II investigators. Use of anastrozole for breast cancer prevention (IBIS-II): long-term results of a randomised controlled trial. Lancet 2020;395(10218):117–22.
84. Noonan S, Pasa A, Fontana V, et al. A survey among breast cancer specialists on the low uptake of therapeutic prevention with tamoxifen or raloxifene. Cancer Prev Res (Phila) 2018;11:38–43.
85. Land SR, Walcott FL, Liu Q, et al. Symptoms and QOL as predictors of chemoprevention adherence in NRG Oncology/NSABP Trial P-1. J Natl Cancer Inst 2015;108:djv365.
86. Ropka ME, Keim J, Philbrick JT. Patient decisions about breast cancer chemoprevention: a systematic review and meta-analysis. J Clin Oncol 2010;28:3090–5.
87. Port ER, Montgomery LL, Heerdt AS, et al. Patient reluctance toward tamoxifen use for breast cancer primary prevention. Ann Surg Oncol 2001;8:580–5.
88. Bambhroliya A, Chavez-MacGregor M, Brewster AM. Barriers to the use of breast cancer risk reduction therapies. J Natl Compr Canc Netw 2015;13:927–35.
89. Brewster AM, Thomas P, Brown P, et al. A System-Level Approach to Improve the Uptake of Antiestrogen Preventive Therapy among Women with Atypical Hyperplasia and Lobular Cancer In Situ. Cancer Prev Res 2018;11(5):295–302.

90. DeCensi A, Puntoni M, Guerrieri-Gonzaga A, et al. Randomized Placebo Controlled Trial of Low-Dose Tamoxifen to Prevent Local and Contralateral Recurrence in Breast Intraepithelial Neoplasia. J Clin Oncol 2019;37(19):1629–37.
91. Taylor LJ, Steiman J, Schumacher JR, et al. Surgical Management of Lobular Carcinoma In Situ: Analysis of the National Cancer Database. Ann Surg Oncol 2018; 25(8):2229–34.
92. Geiger AM, Yu O, Herrinton LJ, et al. A population-based study of bilateral prophylactic mastectomy efficacy in women at elevated risk for breast cancer in community practices. Arch Intern Med 2005;165(5):516–20.
93. Sakurai T, Zhang N, Suzuma T, et al. Long-term follow-up of nipple-sparing mastectomy without radiotherapy: a single center study at a Japanese institution. Med Oncol 2013;30(1):481.
94. Jakub JW, Peled AW, Gray RJ, et al. Oncologic Safety of Prophylactic Nipple-Sparing Mastectomy in a Population With *BRCA* Mutations: A Multi-institutional Study. JAMA Surg 2018;153(2):123–9.
95. Balch C, Klimberg VS, Pawlik T, et al. Textbook of complex general surgical oncology. New York, USA: McGraw-Hill; 2016.

Intraductal Papillomas

Shannon N. Tierney, MD, MS

KEYWORDS

- Papilloma • Intraductal papilloma • Papillary • Breast cancer risk

KEY POINTS

- The risk of intraductal papillomas relates mostly to the risk of undersampling.
- Multiple factors increase the risk of finding malignancy, including the presence of atypia, size, symptoms, and personal risk factors.
- Personalized decision-making is important. Papillomas that are not excised should be observed.

The most common manifestation of papillary breast disease is intraductal papilloma (IDP), which is usually characterized by a pedunculated intraductal mass on a fibrovascular stalk, usually covered by myoepithelial cells creating fronds. Papillary disease also includes papillomatosis (multiple, usually peripherally located papillomas occurring in terminal duct lobular units (TDLUs)), papillary ductal carcinoma *in situ*, encapsulated papillary carcinoma, solid papillary carcinoma, and invasive papillary carcinoma. Intraductal papillomas are considered proliferative disease, which can be associated with a risk ratio for breast cancer of 3.58 without atypia and up to 4.56 with atypia.[1] Furthermore, they fall into the spectrum of "high risk" disease, with an associated risk of upstaging to noninvasive or invasive cancer at excisional biopsy, and potential risk of transformation. However, this designation is controversial, with recent recommendations, announced at the Society of Breast Imagers 2022 symposium (not yet formally adopted), by the ACR BIRADS group to classify papillomas as "benign with upgrade potential" and excision recommended mostly when it is not felt to be adequately sampled.[2] Documentation on pathology reports that the papilloma was felt to be completed excised is reassuring.

When describing this lesion to patients, comparison to a polyp or growth can be helpful, along with the clarification that papillomas of the breast are not associated with HPV. Like polyps, papillomas can hide atypical or malignant cells. Delineating the characteristics of intraductal papillomas which are associated with the risk of upstaging to stratify which papillomas require surgical excision has been challenging, with significant characteristics varying widely from study to study.

Augusta Health Breast Surgery, 70 Medical Center Circle, Suite 107, Fishersville, VA 22939, USA
E-mail address: sntierney@augustahealth.com
Twitter: @SinSeattle75 (S.N.T.)

Surg Clin N Am 102 (2022) 965–972
https://doi.org/10.1016/j.suc.2022.08.011
0039-6109/22/© 2022 Elsevier Inc. All rights reserved.

surgical.theclinics.com

The presentation of papillomas can be clinical or radiological. Papillomas may present with nipple discharge, which is considered pathologic when it is unilateral, spontaneous, and single duct. Associated nipple discharge may be serous or bloody, with bloody discharge coming from friability of the surface epithelium or pedicle torsion creating ischemia. Discharge may also result from associated duct ectasia. Larger and more centrally located papillomas may present as a palpable mass. Radiological presentations depend on imaging modality. Mammograms may show a discrete mass, calcifications, and/or a focal asymmetry. Ultrasound may show a mass, usually but not always appearing to be intraductal, which may be solid, complex solid/cystic, or cystic. These intraductal masses may be associated with a dilated duct, sometimes containing ductal debris, and occasionally may present solely as a dilated duct without a visible mass. MRI most commonly identifies papilloma as an enhancing mass, but may also show only non–mass-like enhancement (NME). (**Figs. 1–3**).

Initial diagnosis is most commonly performed using a core needle biopsy. The use of larger gauge needles, vacuum assistance, and multiple passes has been associated with lower risk of upstaging in multiple studies. In cases with more imaging-occult lesions, use of ductography or ductoscopy has been utilized. With ductography, the duct presenting with discharge is cannulated and radioopaque dye infiltrated into the duct to identify a mass lesion on mammography, which can then be biopsied stereotactically. In ductoscopy, a fine fiberoptic camera is used to visualize the interior of the duct, which can be useful for subtle, sessile papillomas that are centrally located. A ductoscopic basket can even be used to extract papillomas endoscopically, though this has only been described in one published study.[3] Other papillomas may not be diagnosed until surgical excision. If the duct is identifiable at surgery, it can be cannulated with a 0000 lacrimal duct probe or infiltrated with methylene blue so that a selective duct excision can be performed. Alternatively, a central duct excision which excises the subareolar collecting ducts can be performed; as the majority of isolated papillomas are located within 2 cm of the nipple, this will usually capture the offending lesion and eliminates the bothersome symptoms (**Figs. 4 and 5**).

It is generally accepted that symptomatic papillomas be surgically excised. However, the guidelines for surgical excision of asymptomatic papillomas are vague. The American Society of Breast Surgeons Consensus Guidelines recommend excision of papillary lesions with atypia, but suggests that decision on other papillary lesions be individualized using multiple criteria, with close observation using serial imaging as the alternative.[4] When observation is chosen, diagnostic ultrasound at 6, 12, 18, and 24 months in combination with annual mammogram is recommended.[5] This approach is supported by the NHS Breast Screening Programme.[6] The Chinese Society of Breast Surgery recommends excisional biopsy as the first choice for most IDPs, particularly larger lesions or those associated with nipple discharge, though lists vacuum-assisted biopsy as an alternative when the lesion can be fully removed.[7] At

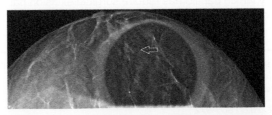

Fig. 1. Large intraductal papilloma (*arrow*) on tomosynthesis mammogram–CC view. (Credit to Brandi Nicholson MD.)

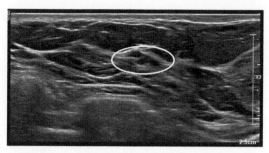

Fig. 2. US appearance of intraductal papilloma (*circle*) with dilated duct. (Credit to Todd Goodnight MD.)

the second International Consensus Conference on B3 lesions, following full removal of the lesions using vacuum-assisted biopsy surveillance without surgical excision was endorsed as acceptable management, based on a malignant upgrade of 7.7% of all 1251 papillary lesions in the Swiss Minimally Invasive Breast Biopsy group data-base.[8] Vacuum-assisted excision, which uses a 7 gauge needle, can remove about 4 g of tissue, reducing the risk of false-negatives even further.[9]

The relevant criteria vary in significance from study to study, making it challenging to create a mental algorithm for surgeons and patients and leading one group to attempt the development of a breast papillary index computational model as a tool for radiol-ogists.[10] In this article, recent large studies evaluating risk factors for upstaging will be reviewed.

PRESENCE OF ATYPIA

The presence of atypia is one of the most significant risk factors for upstaging in most studies. One study evaluated only IDPs without atypia, reviewing 383 lesions that were reviewed again by pathology, showed a very small upgrade risk, with 4.4% upgrading to high-risk atypia and only 0.8% upgrading to malignancy.[11] Another evaluated 500 patients with 206 undergoing surgical excision, and the malignant upgrade rate was

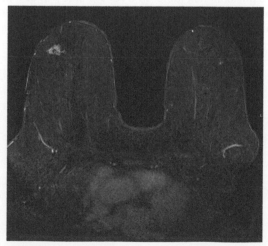

Fig. 3. MRI example of intraductal papilloma with final pathology showing DCIS within the papilloma. (Credit to Brandi Nicholson MD.)

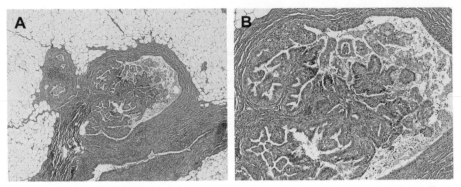

Fig. 4. (*A*). Intraductal papilloma fully removed at core biopsy. (*B*) Intraductal papilloma fully removed at core biopsy–high power. (Credit to Christopher Wenzinger MD.)

only 1.8%.(Choi) In a study of 259 patients comparing IDPs without atypia to those with atypia, a malignant upgrade rate of 7.5% was seen in lesions without atypia but a 30% upgrade was seen in IDPs with atypia or concomittent ADH/ALH.[12] An Australian study of 103 papillary lesions showed a high overall upgrade rate of 30%, representing a 72% upgrade rate in those with atypia and only 7% in those without.[13] Another study of 114 papillary lesions demonstrated upgrade in 47.8% of cases with atypia (22/46) and 13.2% without atypia (9/68).[14]

PALPABLE MASS AND/OR NIPPLE DISCHARGE

Multiple studies have demonstrated a link between presentation with symptoms and upstaging to malignancy. A Chinese retrospective study of 4450 intraductal papillomas in which 51% presented with a palpable mass and 16% presented with both a palpable mass and nipple discharge showed a statistically significant association, with 32% of palpable papillomas showing malignancy on excision compared to 3.4% of nonpalpable papillomas, and 35% of palpable papillomas with discharge showing malignancy compared to 15% of those without.[15] Palpable breast mass was a statistically significant risk factor in a recent study of 327 patients in California.[16] Both palpability and bloody nipple discharge were independent factors in upgrade in a Korean study of 250 patient undergoing open excision of papillary lesions.[17]

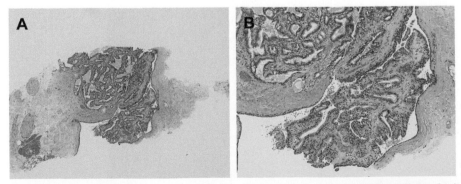

Fig. 5. (*A*). Fragment of intraductal papilloma. (*B*) Fragment of intraductal papilloma–high power. (Credit to Christopher Wenzinger MD.)

HISTORY OF CANCER

Several articles looked at the risk of upstaging in patients with a prior history of breast cancer. One article from Mt. Sinai, reviewing a total of 490 IDPs showed an overall upgrade rate of 12.3% for atypia and 1.1% for cancer.[18] The subgroup of 40 patients with prior breast cancer had a significantly higher risk of upgrade, with 27.5% to atypia (though this would be unlikely to change management) and 5% to new cancer. In MSKCC study of 166 patients where 34.9% had a prior history of breast cancer, 3 of the 4 malignant upgrades were in patients with prior cancer, though this didn't meet statistical significance.[19]

OLDER AGE

The Alberty-Oller study from Mt. Sinai of 490 cases of intraductal papilloma showed a 1.81 prevalence ratio in patients 55 or older, compared with younger patients. Another study of 327 patients showed age greater than 50 was statistically significant.[16] One older study evaluating 205 patients showed that age over 45 was statistically significant.[20]

RACE

While much outcomes data on racial disparities can be attributed to systemic racism, there are some clinical and biological differences among ethnic groups associated with breast cancer, such as ER negativity, high S-phase fraction, and so forth.[21] Few studies have directly examined the effect of race on upgrading of IDPs, but one small study of 29 patients undergoing excision where 25 were African American showed a higher-than-average malignant upgrade rate of 25%, with 2 of 3 patients with IDPs showing atypia upgraded.[22] Further research would be necessary to corroborate this.

SIZE OF PAPILLOMA

Most studies have shown an association between the size of the IDP and risk of upgrade, with 1 cm tending to be the cut-off. A study of 147 patients in Malaysia showed a statistically significant difference in average sonographic size, with benign lesions being a median of 1.0 cm, atypical lesions being a median of 1.1 cm, and malignant lesions being a median of 1.9 cm, though there was overlap with benign lesions as large at 1.35 cm and malignant lesions as small as 0.7 cm.[23] The recent California study of 327 patients showed increased risk of upgrade with size greater than 1.0 cm.[16] An older study of 50 patients also noted that lesions larger than 1 cm tended to have a higher risk of malignancy.[24] A Korean study of 250 lesions after excision showed statistical upgrade when the IDP was > 1.5 cm on imaging.[17] Another study with a low overall upgrade rate of 2.3% also demonstrated statistical correlation with size, showing only 0.9% upgrade for lesions smaller than 1 cm.[25] Size was not, however, a statistical factor in another study of 205 patients, where only atypia and age were relevant.[20] While most studies have looked at sonographic size, MRI size of 1.0 cm or greater was also statistically significant in a logistical regression analysis.[26] This was also seen with mixed mass-non–mass-like enhancement lesions, probably due to the enhancement of adjacent atypical hyperplasia or DCIS or the presence of papillomatosis.

LOCATION IN BREAST

Several studies have suggested that the risk of upgrade to invasive cancer increases with more peripheral locations within the breast, though this is more difficult to characterize. In 327 patients undergoing surgical excision of IDPs demonstrated a significantly increased risk if the lesion was > 5 cm from nipple.[16] Peripheral location was also significant in a study of 250 cases.[17] It has been noted that intraductal papillomas in the axillary tail should also undergo pathological differentiation from rare sweat gland papillary hidradenoma.[27]

NUMBER OF PAPILLOMAS

While the entity of papillomatosis is known to be associated with increased risk for breast cancer, the presence of multiple papillomas in a single patient is also associated with an increased likelihood of upgrading at excision. In Alberty-Oller and colleagues, each additional IDP was associated with a prevalence ratio of 1.51 for overall upgrade and 2.23 PR for malignant upgrade. In the study of 383 IDPs without atypia, multifocality was one of the statistically significant factors for malignant upgrade on univariate analysis, though only 3 cases upgraded.[11]

VASCULARITY

Intralesional vascularity has been shown in some studies to be associated with malignant upgrade, though vascularity is not uncommon due to the fibrovascular core within the feeding pedicle. One study showed vascularity was present in 7/39 cases of benign papillary lesions, and 9/17 cases of malignant papillary lesions, showing overlap.[23]

OVERALL HIGH RISK

A study of 278 patients showed an overall upgrade risk of 14.6%, with a 3.9% upgrade to DCIS.[28] A subgroup of high risk patients, with > 20% lifetime risk of developing breast cancer, was 2.5 times more likely to upgrade.

OTHER

Characteristics that have been evaluated without much statistical association with upgrade include morphology and ductal dilation. Various factors, including margins, echogenicity, posterior features, orientation, echogenic halo, associated calcifications, and architectural distortion have been evaluated, without consistency in statistical significance among studies.

  Management decisions for intraductal papillomas remain challenging, with some contradictory recommendations and lack of clear guidelines. This should be looked at as an opportunity for personalized and shared decision-making, with the goals of balancing surgical risks with the burden of observation, and of determining the goals of treatment, for example, risk stratification due to the presence of atypia at excision, or earliest possible excision vs high likelihood of avoiding the need for surgery. Breast surgeons should be prepared to discuss the nuances to properly inform patient's decision-making.

CLINICS CARE POINTS

- When discussing excision versus observation of IDPs, it is crucial to balance the risks of undersampling with the risks of surgery.
- In patients where upstaging to atypia may not change management and the likelihood of cancer is low, observation may be preferred.

- As atypia can be the strongest predictor for upstaging to cancer, most IDPs with atypia should be excised.

DISCLAIMER

The author has nothing to disclose.

REFERENCES

1. Castells X, Domingo L, Corominas JM, et al. Breast cancer risk after diagnosis by screening mammography of nonproliferative or proliferative benign breast disease: a study from a population-based screening program. Breast Cancer Res Treat 2015;149:237–44.
2. Personal communication, Brandi Nicholson, MD. 6/15/2022.
3. Bender O, Balci FL, Yüney E, et al. Scarless endoscopic papillomectomy of the breast. Onkologie 2009;32:94–8.
4. American Society of Breast Surgeons. Consensus guideline on concordance assessment of image-guided breast biopsies and management of borderline or high-risk lesions. Available at: https://www.breastsurgeons.org/docs/statements/Consensus-Guideline-on-Concordance-Assessment-of-Image-Guided-Breast-Biopsies.pdf?v2. Accessed May 15, 2022.
5. Choi HY, Kim SM, Jang M, et al. Benign Breast Papilloma without Atypia: Outcomes of Surgical Excision versus US-guided Directional Vacuum-assisted Removal or US Follow-up. Radiology 2019;293:72–80.
6. Pinder SE, Shaaban A, Deb R, et al. NHS breast screening multidisciplinary working group guidelines for the diagnosis and management of breast lesions of uncertain malignant potential on core biopsy (B3 lesions). Clin Radiol 2018;73:682–92.
7. Wu D, Shi A, Song A, et al. Clinical practice guidelines for intraductal papilloma: chinese society of breast surgery (CSBrS) practice guidelines 2021. Chin Med J 2021;134:11658–60.
8. Rageth CJ, O'Flynn EAM, Pinker K, et al. Second international consensus conference on lesions of uncertain malignant potential in the breast (B3 lesions). Breast Cancer Res Treat 2019;174:279–96.
9. Catanzariti F, Avendano D, Cicero G, et al. High-risk lesions of the breast:concurrent diagnostic tools and management recommendations. Insights Imaging 2021;12:63.
10. Pham T, Raghavendra U, Koh JEW, et al. Development of breast papillary index for differentiation of benign and malignant lesions using ultrasound images. J Ambient Intelligence Humanized Comput 2021;12:2121–9.
11. Han S, Kim M, Chung YR, et al. Benign intraductal papilloma without atypia on core needle biopsy ahs a low rate of upgrading to malignancy after excision. J Breast Cancer 2018;21:80–6.
12. Khan S, Diaz A, Archer KJ, et al. Papillary lesions of the breast: to excise or observe? Breast J 2017;24:350–5.
13. Armes JE, Galbraith C, Gray J, et al. The outcome of papillary lesions of the breast diagnosed by standard core needle biopsy within a BreastScreen Australia service. Pathology 2017;49:267–70.
14. Bianchi S, Bendinelli B, Saladino V, et al. Non-malignant breast papillary lesions – b3 diagnosed on ultrasound-guided 14-gague needle core biopsy: analysis of

114 cases from a single institution and review of the literature. Pathol Oncol Res 2015;21:535–46.

15. Li X, Wang H, Sun Z, et al. A retrospective observational study of intraductal breast papilloma and its coexisting lesions: a real world experience. Cancer Med 2020;9:77551–762.

16. Kuehner G, Darbinian J, Habel L, et al. Benign papillary breast mass lesions: favorable outcomes with surgical excision or imaging surveillance. Ann Surg Oncol 2019;26:1695–703.

17. Ahn SK, Han W, Moon H, et al. Management of benign papilloma without atypia diagnosed at ultrasound-guided core needle biopsy: scoring system for predicting malignancy. Eur J Surg Oncol 2018;44:53–8.

18. Alberty-Oller JL, Reyes S, Moshier E, et al. Does previous history of cancer or atypia predict histologic upgrade for pure intraductal papillomas diagnosed via core biopsy? A study of 490 cases at a single institution. Cancer Rep 2022;5:e1481.

19. Pareja F, Corben A, Brennan S, et al. Breast intraductal papillomas without atypia in radiologic-pathologic concordant core needle biopsys: predictors of upgrade to carcinoma at excision. Cancer 2016;122:2819–27.

20. Cheng T, Chen C, Lee M, et al. Risk factors associated with conversion from nonmalignant to malignant diagnosis after surgical excision of breast papillary lesions. Ann Surg Oncol 2009;16:3375–9.

21. Brawley OW. Health disparities in breast cancer. Obstet Gynecol Clin M Am 2013; 40:513–23.

22. Wang H, Tsang PD, Cruz C, et al. Follow-up of breast papillary lesion on core needle biopsy: experience in African-American population. Diagn Pathol 2014;9:86.

23. Fadzli F, Rhamat K, Ramli MT, et al. Spectrum of imaging findings of papillary breast disease – A radiopathyological review in a tertiary center. Medicine 2021;100:16.

24. Kuzmiak C, Lewis M, Zeng D, et al. Role of sonography in the differentiation of benign, high-risk, and malignancy papillary lesions of the breast. J Ultrasound Med 2014;33:1545–52.

25. Ko d, Kang E, Park SY, et al. The management strategy of benign solitary intraductal papilloma on breast core biopsy. Clin Breast Cancer 2017;17:367–72.

26. Wang L, Wu P, Li X, et al. Magnetic resonance imaging features for differentiating breast papilloma with high-risk or malignant lesions from benign papilloma: a retrospective study on 158 patients. World J Surg Oncol 2018;16:234.

27. Kulka J, Madaras L, Floris G. Papillary lesions of the breast. Virchows Archive 2022;480:1.

28. Chen Y, Mack J, Karamchandani D, et al. Excision recommended in high-risk patients: revisiting the diagnosis of papilloma on core biopsy in the context of patient risk. Breast J 2019;25:232–6.

Management of Common Complications of Lactation
The Breast Surgeon's Role in Examining the Science and Debunking Old Myths

Katrina B. Mitchell, MD, IBCLC[a],*, Helen M. Johnson, MD, IBCLC[b]

KEYWORDS

- Lactation • Breastfeeding • Mastitis • Breast abscess • Galactocele • Milk fistula
- Nipple bleb

KEY POINTS

- Breast surgeons are well poised to promote evidence-based recommendations for lactation-related breast disorders.
- Milk fistula is an uncommon complication of invasive procedures and is best managed with continued breastfeeding.
- To avoid the need for repeat aspirations, lactational abscesses and infected galactoceles may be drained with a stab incision and percutaneous drain insertion at bedside.
- Lactation-related nipple wounds should be treated with closed, moist wound healing.
- "Plugging" represents ductal inflammation rather than macroscopic obstruction, and lactational mastitis is more often inflammatory than infectious.
- Fungal infections do not contribute to breast and nipple pain during lactation.

INTRODUCTION

Although lactation consultants traditionally have assumed care of breastfeeding mothers, many women require thorough evaluation and treatment by physicians, which may involve diagnostic evaluation of medical conditions, prescribing antibiotics, or performing invasive procedures such as abscess drainage. Despite the complexity of lactation as a physiologic process and challenges in caring for these patients, lactation education in medical school and residency is extremely limited.

Funding: none.
[a] Department of Surgical Oncology, Ridley-Tree Cancer Center, Sansum Clinic, 540 West Pueblo Street, Santa Barbara, CA 93105, USA; [b] Department of Surgery, Brody School of Medicine, East Carolina University, 600 Moye Boulevard, Greenville, NC 27834, USA
* Corresponding author.
E-mail address: kbm9002@me.com

Breast surgeons possess intimate knowledge of breast anatomy and physiology and regularly interface with breast pathology and radiology. Therefore, they are in a unique position to recognize and reframe traditional breastfeeding recommendations that may be flawed. Surgeons also can provide insight into appropriate wound care for conditions such as nipple trauma and perform invasive procedures such as drainage of fluid collections. This article reviews common management approaches for complications of lactation applicable to surgical practices.

MILK FISTULA
Myth

Procedures should be avoided on the lactating breast due to the risk of milk fistula.

Science

Milk fistula is rare if lactation and surgical interventions are managed appropriately.[1,2] After a procedure, patients should not avoid breastfeeding. In fact, the preferential flow of breastmilk through the nipple will decrease the flow through a needle or incision tract. On the other hand, patients should not be counseled to "pump to empty" their breasts or breastfeed more frequently on the affected breast, as this will cause increase in milk production, which will promote fistula persistence.

Treatment

Large surgical incision and drainage should be avoided in lactation patients. Any incision made should be as small as possible, and as distant from the nipple areolar complex as possible. If a distal incision is not possible, it should be made outside the region where an infant latches or pump flanges contact the skin. Periareolar incisions, although cosmetic, are particularly high risk due to the potential for latch or pump trauma.

Patients should feed physiologically after a procedure. Local anesthetic agents are not absorbed orally by the infant, and blood is safe for the infant to ingest.[3] A transient fistula will form after any procedure but is expected to close within a week if lactation is managed appropriately.

Should a persistent, high-output fistula develop, a distal diverting drain can be placed to hasten closure[1] (**Fig. 1**). Milk passing through a fistula tract may be collected and is safe to feed to the infant.[4] Absorbent dressings may be used to prevent skin maceration from moisture but should be removed before breastfeeding, as they are potential choking hazards and/or may interfere with latch. Wound vacuum systems should not be used on the lactating breast, as this will promote chronic fistulization and maintain tract patency.

DRAINAGE OF ABSCESS AND GALACTOCELE
Myth

Fluid collections in the lactating breast require operative incision and drainage or aspiration alone.

Science

As surgeons have moved away from large incision and drainage procedures performed on the lactating breast in the operating room setting, they have turned to minimally invasive aspiration approach.[5] However, aspiration alone can result in incomplete drainage.[6] Unlike simple breast cysts, abscesses and galactoceles in the lactating breast contain breastmilk, which is highly viscous and loculated

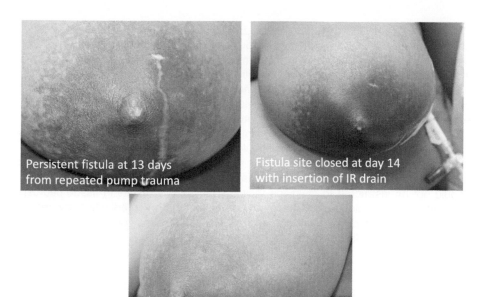

Fig. 1. Transient milk fistula in setting of hyperlactation and pump trauma, located near nipple areolar complex with resolution 24 hours after placement of distal diverting Interventional Radiology (IR) drain.

(**Fig. 2**). Therefore, a needle aspiration alone will likely remove only part of the fluid collection, particularly if it is chronic. If a needle aspiration *is* successful in removing the entire volume of an acute collection, the area can refill with milk very quickly and require repeated procedures.[7]

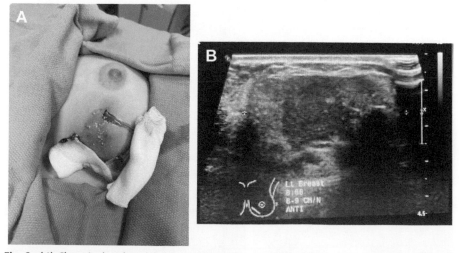

Fig. 2. (*A*) Chronic, loculated fluid collection demonstrating thick milk chunks at definitive drainage after needle aspiration failed to resolve. (*B*) Ultrasound image corresponding to semisolid appearance of the collection.

Treatment

Lactational abscess and infected galactocele require drainage for source control. Drainage may also be appropriate for symptomatic noninfected galactoceles. Small stab incision and drain placement will definitively resolve fluid collections in the lactating breast.[8] The small stab incision allows for access to the cavity with an instrument that can be used to disrupt loculations and provide complete drainage, such as a hemostat. A stent or drain can be placed to allow passive decompression of the area for 3 to 5 days; this could involve a Penrose drain, Seromacath, Blake drain, or other wicks such as a small foley catheter. Drains should be placed to gravity rather than suction.

In addition to the surgical management, many patients developing fluid collections during lactation require treatment of idiopathic or iatrogenic hyperlactation. Patients should not be instructed to massage their breast, as this results in tissue necrosis and phlegmon development.[9–13] Ice and antiinflammatory medication by mouth should be recommended for symptomatic relief. Antibiotics may be indicated if significant surrounding cellulitis exists.

MASTITIS
Myth

Mastitis represents a bacterial infection resulting from milk stasis, engorgement, and "plugging."

Science

When an infant sleeps through the night or mothers do not express their milk at work as regularly as the infant breastfeeds at home, patients experience transient engorgement and pain. Women may also develop breast erythema and edema from congested capillaries and interstitial fluid (**Fig. 3**), which can cause sweating, fever, and chills, as it is an inflammatory process in a body organ with robust blood supply. This systemic inflammatory response syndrome may be mistaken for signs and symptoms of infection, raising alarm for impending development of bacterial mastitis.[10] However, unless a

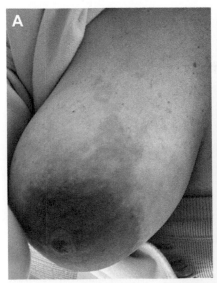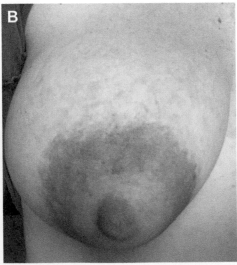

Fig. 3. Acute inflammatory mastitis (A) managed with decreased removal of breastmilk, ice, and antiinflammatory medication, with resolution of erythema (B).

person has developed a very rare rapidly progressive soft tissue infection, it is otherwise very unusual for average bacterial mastitis to present this quickly.

Lactation literature commonly describes a theory that mastitis results from milk stasis. Mothers are warned to avoid long stretches without breastfeeding or pumping to avoid build-up of stagnant milk and progression to "plugging" and infectious mastitis. However, there is no scientific evidence to support the idea that mastitis results from milk stasis. In contrast to a passive repository such as a bladder, the breast is a gland with production regulated by Feedback Inhibitor of Lactation (FIL). Therefore, continued removal of milk increases production and worsens tissue edema and inflammation. Reduced removal of milk will allow for FIL to downregulate production and enable resorption of milk not used.

Mastitis results from underlying microbiome disruption and ductal inflammation[11] and is therefore often observed in patients with hyperlactation and/or blebs. Most cases of lactational mastitis are purely inflammatory and can be resolved with conservative measures and appropriate management of lactation. Breastmilk contains numerous immunologic cells and substances that counteract infection. In similar fashion, it is uncommon for stagnant milk contained in a galactocele to become infected without an inciting event such as instrumentation.

It also should be noted that external compression by a bra or tight clothing can obstruct ducts is not scientifically founded.

Treatment

With early inflammatory mastitis, patients should feed physiologically (eg, eliminate breast pump usage if possible, and do not continue "overfeeding" on the affected breast). Reducing overstimulation of an engorged or inflamed breast will allow downregulation of milk production through the FIL receptor.[12] Patients should never be counseled to "pump to relieve engorgement" as this prevents FIL from activating and perpetuates hyperlactation.

Patients can use ice and antiinflammatory medication by mouth such as nonsteroidal antiinflammatory drugs and/or obtain pain relief from acetaminophen. Ice is generally the most helpful, but some people also prefer heat for comfort. Therapeutic ultrasound can use thermal energy to reduce inflammation and pain, as can lymphatic drainage.[13] A supportive bra is necessary during lactation to prevent dependent lymphedema and back pain. Massage should be strictly avoided. If symptoms persist or worsen, antibiotics should be considered[14] (Table 1). Women should be counseled that there is no medical indication to "pump and dump" while taking these antibiotics. The Relative Infant Dose (RID) estimates an infant's exposure to a medication through breastmilk and depends on multiple factors including the medication's plasma concentration, half-life, solubility, and oral bioavailability. In general, medications with RID less than 10% are considered safe.

MASSAGE
Myth

"Plugging" represents occlusion of ducts by stagnant milk, and "plugs" should be extruded through massage.

Science

The sensation of "plugging" does not represent discrete collections of breastmilk. More accurately, a "plug" represents a focal area of congested capillaries, distended alveolar cells, and tissue edema. The root cause of "plugging" relates to tissue

Table 1
Antibiotics for infectious mastitis

Antibiotic	Dosage	Special Considerations	Relative Infant Dose (RID)[a]
Dicloxacillin, flucloxacillin	500 mg four times a day for 10–14 d		0.6%–1.4%
Cephalexin	500 mg four times a day for 10–14 d	Gram-negative rod coverage	0.4%–1.5%
Clindamycin	300 mg four times a day for 10–14 d	MRSA coverage	0.9%–1.8%
Trimethoprim-sulfamethoxazole	Double strength (160 mg-800 mg) twice a day for 10–14 d	MRSA coverage; contraindicated in G6PD deficiency; caution in premature infants and newborns <30 day old	Trimethoprim: 3.9%–9.9% Sulfamethoxazole: 2.1%–3.1%

Abbreviation: MRSA, methicillin-resistant *Staphylococcus aureus.*
[a] Data from InfantRisk Center, Texas Tech University Health Sciences Center.

hypervascularity, edema, and ductal narrowing from microbiome changes and luminal inflammation.[15]

Lactation consultants often recommend massage for "plugs." However, this recommendation lacks scientific validity and causes tissue trauma that can result in significant complications. As surgeons are well aware, lactating breasts have robust blood supply, lymphatic vessels to drain increased interstitial fluid during lactation, nerves, fibroadipose tissue, and functional glandular tissue with a complex network of interlacing ducts. Attempts to extrude a milk "plug" from a duct with aggressive massage will result in tissue trauma, edema, collapse of ducts, and capillary damage. All patients report worsened pain with massage. As we would injure a thyroid, pancreas, or other functional gland with massage or tissue mishandling during a surgical procedure, it similarly must be avoided in the lactating breast. Massage is associated with development of lactational phlegmon (**Fig. 4**), particularly in the setting of hyperlactation or excessive pumping.[9]

Treatment

Deep manual massage, vibrators, electric toothbrushes, or any commercial breast massage products designed to extrude a "plug" should be strictly avoided. Patients with symptomatic "plugging" should be evaluated for proinflammatory conditions such as hyperlactation and subacute mastitis. Patients can use ice for both pain relief and vasoconstriction. Therapeutic ultrasound, also used to treat conditions such as radiation fibrosis, can reduce inflammation and pain through application of thermal energy (**Fig. 5**).[16] If a mass or erythema persists, diagnostic breast imaging should be performed.[17]

NIPPLE WOUND CARE IN LACTATION
Myth

Nipple wounds in lactating women should be treated with drying agents and topical antibiotics to prevent progression to mastitis.

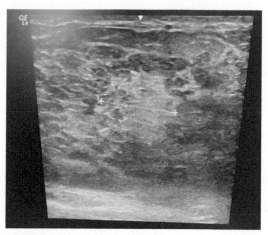

Fig. 4. Ultrasound image of inflammatory phlegmon.

Science

Surgical training provides strong education in wound care techniques and teaches the difference between traumatized versus infected tissue. Surgeons debride devitalized tissue and understand the need to provide absorption for serous fluid and fibrinous exudate. However, traditional lactation recommendations have contradicted principles of closed, moist healing for wound care. Patients are often counseled to express a small amount of breastmilk onto nipple wounds and allow it to air dry. They also may be recommended to soak nipples in Epsom salt or salt water and to use a hair dryer to prevent moisture build-up. They are also often instructed to avoid wearing a bra or allow anything touch the nipples.

In addition, breastfeeding patients with nipple wounds are often warned they are at risk for ascending intraductal infection, that is, bacterial mastitis. They are therefore encouraged to apply topical antibiotics to their wounds. However, it is very uncommon for open, vascularized wounds to become secondarily infected in immunocompetent hosts. Overutilization of antibiotics contributes to disruption of the microbiome and development of multidrug-resistant pathogens. Routine use of topical antibiotics for open wounds is not recommended.[18] Furthermore, the hypothesis that bacterial mastitis is a result of ascending infection from nipple wounds is not supported by

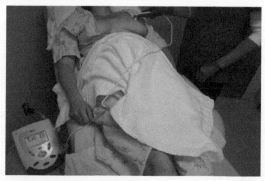

Fig. 5. Therapeutic ultrasound technique.

breast anatomy and physiology.[19] The highly vascular nature of the lactating breast and the multiple immune components of breastmilk prevent such infection.[8]

Treatment

Care of the nipples is summarized in **Box 1**.

FUNGAL INFECTIONS

Myth

Yeast is a common cause of nipple and breast pain and infections in lactating women.

Science

Although the lactation world for decades has implicated yeast as a causative agent in symptomatology of pain, redness, and/or itching of the nipple and breast, there is no scientific evidence to support this claim.[15] New reports demonstrate the mis- and overdiagnosis of this condition.[20]

Symptomatic fungal infections result from host-microbiome disruption and occur most commonly in the vaginal mucosa or in the inframammary region of the breast. Yeast infections also may occur in skin folds of patients with morbid obesity and in patients with immunosuppression (eg, diabetes, immunologic disorders such as human immunodeficiency virus/AIDS, or in the setting of chemotherapy). Although yeast is ubiquitous in normal skin flora, pathogenic infections of the nipple and breast in immunocompetent individuals are extremely uncommon. The lactating nipple has robust blood supply, and breastmilk has multiple antibacterial properties, making epidermal and deep soft tissue infections rare.

Patients may believe they improve after antifungal treatment; this is related to the antiinflammatory effect some people obtain from antifungals or the fact they removed a contact allergen they had been using (eg, nipple balm containing lanolin). However, the improvement is almost always not definitive, and patients will return for repeat treatment or seek alternative interventions.

Breastfeeding women whose infants are diagnosed with thrush are often advised that they are at risk for yeast infections of the nipple and breast. They are instructed to take antifungals and sterilize bottles and breast pump parts to prevent infection. However, thrush is not contagious. More importantly, infant thrush in full-term, immunocompetent babies is not nearly as common as the lactation world describes. Many babies simply have a white coating on their tongue and/or cheeks from normal breastmilk.

Treatment

Evaluate for common cause of nipple irritation and pain, including trauma, nipple blebs, vasospasm, hyperesthesia, and dermatitis. Patients with nipple trauma require closed, moist wound healing. Patients with symptomatic blebs should be treated with a medium-potency steroid such as 0.1% triamcinolone.[21] Vasospasm and hyperesthesia resolve with constant warmth (wool pads and other insulating bra liners, heating pads, and so forth) and/or the selective serotonin reuptake inhibitor class of drugs.[22,23] A diagnosis of dermatitis requires determination of the inciting agent and its discontinuation, as well as a short course of topical steroid (**Fig. 8**).[24] Atypical dermatitis and dermatitis that does not respond to appropriate therapy should raise concern for Paget disease of the nipple and be evaluated with diagnostic breast imaging and biopsies.

When infants undergo thrush treatment, mothers do not need to undergo antifungal treatment themselves. Topical and oral antifungals are not indicated in lactation.

Box 1
Clinics care points: care of the nipples during lactation

- Moist, closed wound healing principles should be followed, with the use of nonallergenic ointments/balms and sterile, absorbent dressings **(Fig. 6)**.

- Avoid ointments/balms containing potentially allergenic ingredients such as lanolin and petroleum.

- APNO (All Purpose Nipple Ointment) should be avoided. This compounded prescription ointment contains an antifungal, antibacterial, and a steroid. Although often recommended by lactation consultants and readily prescribed by the physicians to whom patients are referred, this nonspecific medication can cause additional complications. Although patients may achieve some pain relief due to steroids and antiinflammatory properties of the antifungal, this potential benefit is outweighed by the risks of impaired wound healing from steroids and of microbiome disruption from nonselective elimination of normal flora. Furthermore, other ingredients in this ointment may cause dermatitis. This medication is generally expensive, even for patients with insurance.

- Breast shells designed to "keep the nipple dry" or "protect the nipple from the bra" worsen swelling in the nipple, cause areola compression, and subsequently worsen pain.

- Do not use drying agents such as antiseptics, alcohol, or Epsom salt soaks **(Fig. 7)**. Similarly, do not use a hair dryer to blow hot, dehumidified air on nipples. These practices cause tissue desiccation, which is counterproductive for wound healing and increase the risk of skin breakdown.

Antifungal creams and ointments applied to the nipple or to the mouth of the baby can be very irritating to the nipple and areola, worsening vasospasm and causing surface wounds from contact dermatitis. Gentian violet can cause nipple ulceration and mouth ulceration in a baby and should not be used.[25] Pump parts, infant toys, and other household items do not need to be sterilized; in fact, harsh detergents may worsen epidermal barrier breakdown and allergy, which is often at the root of the mother's symptomatology.

NIPPLE BLEBS
Myth

Nipple blebs are caused by trauma from shallow infant latch.

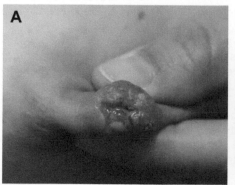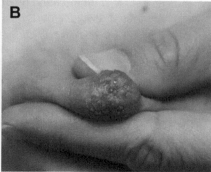

Fig. 6. Nipple previously air dried (*A*), with resolution of tissue defect with PolyMem therapy (*B*).

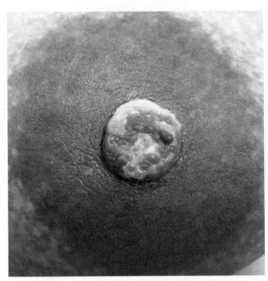

Fig. 7. Blistering from small pump flanges worsened with Epsom salt soaks.

Science

Blebs appear as small white, yellow, or red blisterlike lesions on the surface of a nipple. They are inflammatory lesions that may occlude a nipple orifice. They reflect underlying ductal inflammation and microbiome disruption with biofilm formation.[21] Blebs are associated with hyperlactation (oversupply), pumping (which alters the breast microbiome), c-section births (which also alter the breast microbiome), and other characteristics of individual variation in microbiome expression.[26] Blebs are not related to infant trauma or latch in any way. Because blebs are very painful, moms often believe the infant has a poor latch or otherwise has contributed to the problem. However, this represents an association rather than causation.

Treatment

Asymptomatic blebs do not require any specific treatment. Blebs causing milk obstruction warrant treatment to reduce underlying ductal inflammation and decrease the viscosity of milk. Sunflower lecithin by mouth is effective for breastmilk emulsification and can help to both treat and prevent blebs.[21] Therapeutic ultrasound can also be used to reduce breast inflammation.

Symptomatic blebs occluding an orifice should be treated with oral lecithin as well as a topical medium-potency steroid such as 0.1% triamcinolone cream.[21] Blebs should not be routinely unroofed with a sterile needle or other means, as this may transiently relieve milk obstruction in an associated ductal orifice but will also cause local tissue trauma and can lead to scarring (**Fig. 9**).[27] This scarring can result in permanent occlusion of the nipple orifice. Patients should be instructed not to attempt to squeeze out a bleb or pick at it with their fingernails, as this can cause bleeding and further trauma.

NIPPLE/AREOLAR LESIONS AND PIERCINGS
Myth

Women with nipple/areolar lesions and nipple piercings should be discouraged from breastfeeding.

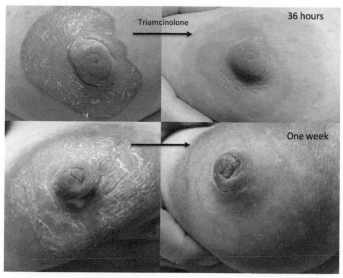

Fig. 8. Two patients with contact dermatitis worsened by caustic antifungal agents with resolution after treatment with topical steroids.

Science

Several lesions can occur on the nipple/areolar complex including nipple adenomas, skin tags, eczema, and hyperkeratosis. Patients with these conditions are often advised to avoid breastfeeding due to concerns about latch and milk extraction, as well as theoretic risks of an infant choking on a protruding lesion or suffering toxicity from medications used to treat dermatologic conditions.

Patients with nipple piercings may be advised to avoid breastfeeding altogether due to concerns about milk fistulae. Milk will indeed pass through the piercing sites (**Fig. 10**); however, this does not negatively affect milk production or extraction, nor does it pose a risk to the mother's health in any way.

Treatment

Women with nipple/areolar lesions should be evaluated by a breastfeeding medicine physician prenatally. These physicians may recommend removal of larger lesions if they are concerned about interference with latch or potential for tissue trauma. Surgical excision can be performed under local anesthesia during pregnancy or lactation with minimal risk.

In most of the cases, prenatal evaluation of nipple/areolar lesions will consist of review of the lactational safety of medications and reassurance. Topical steroids, keratolytic ointments, and most immunomodulators used for conditions such as eczema, psoriasis, and hyperkeratosis are safe in lactation, with the exception of methotrexate.[27] Nipple shields should not be recommended to cover nipple/areolar complex lesions, as there is no benefit to this practice and nipple shields are associated with decreased physiologic milk transfer and increased risk of microbiome disruption and mastitis.[28]

Ideally, patients should remove nipple piercings during early pregnancy, as the nipple is expected to hypertrophy and can make later removal more difficult. Nipple piercings are a choking hazard, and patients should not breastfeed with them.

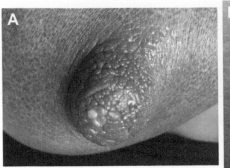
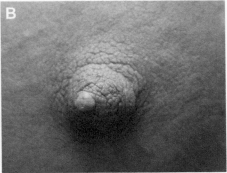

Fig. 9. Nipple bleb at presentation (*A*) and after chronic tissue trauma from frequent unroofing (*B*).

When consenting for piercings, women should be counseled that the procedure may result in ductal trauma or scarring that could impair lactation.

INVERTED OR FLAT NIPPLES
Myth

Women with inverted or flat nipples should perform nipple eversion exercises during the prenatal period.

Science

Up to 10% of the female population has inverted or flat-appearing nipples.[19] However, this anatomic variant uncommonly precludes lactation if managed appropriately. In fact, in many cases, the tissue bands tethering the nipple in the inverted position are released by the mechanics of breastfeeding or pumping (**Fig. 11**).[27] Prenatal exercises to evert the nipples using a designated suction device or nipple shells have not been shown to improve lactation outcomes.[29] In fact, some studies suggest that these exercises have a negative impact on a mother's desire to attempt breastfeeding.[30]

Treatment

Infants may latch without issue to an inverted nipple. Others may struggle. Performing manual eversion or briefly using a pump before nursing may facilitate infant latch to the stimulus of an erect nipple. Patients with significantly inverted nipples that cannot be

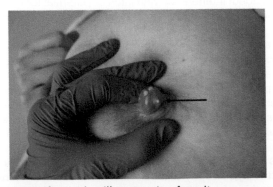

Fig. 10. Nipple piercing orifice with milk emanating from it.

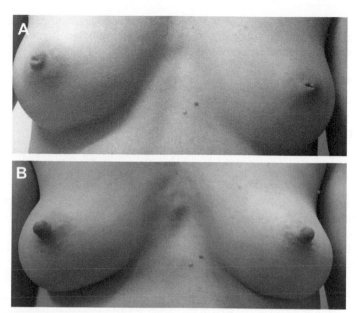

Fig. 11. Patient with nipple slit inversions during pregnancy (*A*) with everted nipples after breastfeeding and pumping (*B*).

manually everted on examination may experience the most challenges. They should not be counseled to perform prenatal exercises.

Women with inverted or flat nipples seeking cosmetic surgery should be counseled about the risk of impaired lactation and advised to defer this procedure until childbearing and breastfeeding are complete. Not only does this surgery sever the terminal ducts resulting in outflow obstruction but it may also disrupt nipple innervation and vasculature. Women with a history of nipple eversion surgery who wish to breastfeed should be referred for prenatal lactation counseling to discuss the potential for impaired lactation, and their newborns should be closely monitored for weight gain and hydration. Recommendations for donor breastmilk and/or formula can be provided if necessary.

SUMMARY

Using their knowledge of breast physiology, histology, and anatomy, surgeons are well equipped to manage challenging complications of breastfeeding, as well as reframe myths in traditional lactation care. Surgeons should recognize that a procedure may result in a transient milk fistula, and both abrupt cessation of breastfeeding and hyperlactation can perpetuate fistula persistence. Needle aspiration of a loculated lactational fluid collection may fail to resolve symptoms without repeated intervention; therefore, a small drain placement at index procedure represents optimal management. Mastitis should be managed by treating hyperlactation, avoiding massage, and using antiinflammatories and ice before antibiotics. Appropriate techniques of closed, moist wound healing should be applied for nipple trauma. Fungal infections of the nipple and breast parenchyma are extraordinarily rare, and common diagnoses such as dermatitis should be explored. Blebs are inflammatory lesions related to ductal microbiome disruption that present on the surface of the nipple, and unroofing should be avoided. Nipple areolar complex masses, conditions, and/or piercings do not preclude breastfeeding, but patients should be evaluated prenatally to guide appropriate management.

DISCLOSURE

The Authors have no commercial or financial conflicts of interest.

REFERENCES

1. Johnson HM, Mitchell KB. Low incidence of milk fistula with continued breast-feeding following radiologic and surgical interventions on the lactating breast. Breast Dis 2021;40(3):183–9.
2. Dominici LS, Kuerer HM, Babiera G, et al. Wound complications from surgery in pregnancy-associated breast cancer (PABC). Breast Dis 2010;31(1):1–5.
3. LactMed. (Drugs and lactation database) lidocaine. National Library of Medicine (US); 2020. Available at: https://www.ncbi.nlm.nih.gov/books/NBK501230/. Accessed February 26, 2022.
4. Barker P. Milk fistula: an unusual complication of breast biopsy. J R Coll Surg Edinb 1988;33(2):106.
5. Irusen H, Rohwer AC, Steyn DW, et al. Treatments for breast abscesses in breastfeeding women. Cochrane Database Syst Rev 2015;(8):CD010490.
6. Li Y, Ma XJ. Risk factors for failure of ultrasound-guided fine-needle aspiration therapy for lactational breast abscess. Breastfeed Med 2021;16(11):894–8.
7. Valente SA, Grobmyer SR. Mastitis and Breast Abscess. In: Bland KI, Copeland EM, Klimberg VS, et al, editors. The breast: comprehensive management of benign and malignant diseases. 5th edition. Elsevier; 2018. p. 93–103, e2:chap 6.
8. Mitchell KB, Johnson HM. Challenges in the management of breast conditions during lactation. Obstet Gynecol Clin North Am 2022;49(1):35–55.
9. Johnson HM, Mitchell KB. Lactational phlegmon: a distinct clinical entity affecting breastfeeding women within the mastitis-abscess spectrum. Breast J 2019. https://doi.org/10.1111/tbj.13624.
10. Kujawa-Myles S, Noel-Weiss J, Dunn S, et al. Maternal intravenous fluids and postpartum breast changes: a pilot observational study. Int Breastfeed J 2015; 10:18.
11. Rodríguez J, Fernández L. Infectious mastitis during lactation: a mammary dysbiosis model. In: McGuire M, McGuire M, Bode L, editors. Prebiotics and probiotics in human milk. Academic Press; 2017. p. 401–28.
12. Weaver SR, Hernandez LL. Autocrine-paracrine regulation of the mammary gland. J Dairy Sci 2016;99(1):842–53.
13. Lavigne V, Gleberzon BJ. Ultrasound as a treatment of mammary blocked duct among 25 postpartum lactating women: a retrospective case series. J Chiropr Med 2012;11(3):170–8.
14. WHO. Mastitis: Causes and Management. Publication Number WHO/FCH/CAH/00.13. 2000.
15. Jimenez E, Arroyo R, Cardenas N, et al. Mammary candidiasis: A medical condition without scientific evidence? PLoS One 2017;12(7):e0181071.
16. Mogensen N, Portman A, Mitchell K. Nonpharmacologic approaches to pain, engorgement, and plugging in lactation: applying physical therapy techniques from breast cancer care to breastfeeding patients. Clin Lactation 2020;11(1).

17. Mitchell KB, Johnson HM, Eglash A. ABM clinical protocol #30: breast masses, breast complaints, and diagnostic breast imaging in the lactating woman. Breastfeed Med 2019;14(4):208–14.
18. Coldiron BM, Fischoff RM, AAo Dermatology. American Academy of Dermatology Choosing Wisely List: helping dermatologists and their patients make smart decisions about their care and treatment. J Am Acad Dermatol 2013;69(6):1002.
19. Stone K, Wheeler A. A Review of Anatomy, Physiology, and Benign Pathology of the Nipple. Ann Surg Oncol 2015;22(10):3236–40.
20. Betts RC, Johnson HM, Eglash A, et al. It's Not Yeast: Retrospective Cohort Study of Lactating Women with Persistent Nipple and Breast Pain. Breastfeed Med 2021;16(4):318–24.
21. Mitchell KB, Johnson HM. Breast Pathology That Contributes to Dysfunction of Human Lactation: a Spotlight on Nipple Blebs. J Mammary Gland Biol Neoplasia 2020;25(2):79–83.
22. Anderson JE, Held N, Wright K. Raynaud's phenomenon of the nipple: a treatable cause of painful breastfeeding. Pediatrics 2004;113(4):e360–4.
23. Berens P, Eglash A, Malloy M, et al. ABM clinical protocol #26: persistent pain with breastfeeding. Breastfeed Med 2016;11(2):46–53.
24. Barrett ME, Heller MM, Fullerton Stone H, et al. Dermatoses of the breast in lactation. Dermatol Ther 2013;26(4):331–6.
25. Utter AR. Gentian violet treatment for thrush: can its use cause breastfeeding problems? J Hum Lact 1990;6(4):178–80.
26. Mitchell KB, Eglash A, Bamberger ET. Mammary Dysbiosis and Nipple Blebs Treated With Intravenous Daptomycin and Dalbavancin. J Hum Lact 2019. https://doi.org/10.1177/0890334419862214. 890334419862214.
27. Mitchell K, Johnson H. Breast Conditions in the Breastfeeding Mother. In: Lawrence R, Lawrence R, editors. Breastfeeding: a guide for the medical profession. 9 edition. Elsevier; 2021. p. 572–93.
28. McKechnie AC, Eglash A. Nipple shields: a review of the literature. Breastfeed Med 2010;5(6):309–14.
29. Preparing for breast feeding: treatment of inverted and non-protractile nipples in pregnancy. The MAIN Trial Collaborative Group. Midwifery 1994;10(4):200–14.
30. Alexander JM, Grant AM, Campbell MJ. Randomised controlled trial of breast shells and Hoffman's exercises for inverted and non-protractile nipples. BMJ 1992;304(6833):1030–2.

19. Mitchell KB, Johnson HM, Eglash A. ABM clinical protocol #30: breast masses, breast complaints, and diagnostic breast imaging in the lactating woman. Breast Feed Med 2019;14(4):208–14.

20. Coulter EM, Lodhi IP. AAP Committee. A new on...

Management of Gynecomastia and Male Benign Diseases

Manish M. Karamchandani, MD[a], Gabriel De La Cruz Ku, MD[b,c], Bradford L. Sokol, BS[d], Abhishek Chatterjee, MD MBA[e], Christopher Homsy, MD[e,*]

KEYWORDS

- Gynecomastia • Benign male breast disease • Pseudogynecomastia • Lipomastia

KEY POINTS

- Gynecomastia is a relatively common benign male breast disease that is often self-limiting.
- Workup begins with a thorough history and physical, as well as a comprehensive metabolic workup to rule out cancer or other pathologic conditions.
- Management of gynecomastia begins with removal of possible offending agents, followed by androgen deprivation therapy.
- If medical management fails, surgical management involving one of several breast reduction techniques can be used.
- Surgical management of gynecomastia is most effective in patients with refractory disease.

GYNECOMASTIA
Definition

Gynecomastia is the benign enlargement of male breast due to increased proliferation of glandular tissue (ie, ductal hyperplasia).[1,2] Gynecomastia should be differentiated from pseudogynecomastia (lipomastia), which is an enlargement of the male breast due to adipose tissue hypertrophy, without glandular involvement.[1,2] Gynecomastia is thought to develop in response to a hormonal shift in the balance between estrogens and androgens that favors a relative increase in estrogens.[1-3] The causes of the

[a] Department of Surgery, Tufts Medical Center; [b] Department of Surgery, UMass Memorial Medical Center; [c] Universidad Científica del Sur, Lima, Peru; [d] Tufts University School of Medicine; [e] Division of Plastic and Reconstructive Surgery, Tufts Medical Center, 800Washington Street, Boston, MA 02111, USA
* Corresponding author.
E-mail address: chomsy@tuftsmedicalcenter.org

Surg Clin N Am 102 (2022) 989–1005
https://doi.org/10.1016/j.suc.2022.06.003
0039-6109/22/© 2022 Elsevier Inc. All rights reserved.

hormonal flux seen in gynecomastia are highly variable and may be physiologic or pathologic in nature.

Epidemiology

Physiologic gynecomastia is generally observed in 3 distinct age groups within the larger male population: neonates, adolescents, and older adults. Neonatal gynecomastia is thought to be the result of exposure to high concentrations of maternal estrogens and is observed in 60% to 90% of the newborn male population.[2,4] Neonatal gynecomastia is typically self-limiting, resolving within 2 to 3 weeks after delivery.[4]

Pubertal gynecomastia is estimated to have a prevalence anywhere between 22% and 69% in adolescent boys with most cases occurring between ages 13 and 14 after the onset of testicular development.[4–7] Lack of consistency regarding the size of palpable glandular tissue required for diagnosis may explain the wide range in reported prevalence among adolescents.[2,8] Approximately 95% to 97% of pubertal gynecomastia cases will resolve without treatment within 18 months of initial discovery.[1,4] Persistent pubertal gynecomastia accounts for approximately 25% of all cases of gynecomastia.[9]

Gynecomastia in older adults is highly prevalent and may affect as many as 36% to 57% of men in this age group.[4,10–12] Unlike children and younger adults, gynecomastia in older adults is more associated with pathologic causes. Pathologic gynecomastia has been linked to numerous pathologic conditions including cirrhosis, malnutrition, drugs, hypogonadism, testicular tumors, hyperthyroidism, and chronic kidney disease.[1,2] Approximately 58% of all cases of adult gynecomastia are idiopathic.[2,9]

Pathophysiology

The basic underlying mechanism responsible for the proliferation of glandular tissue in the breast is commonly thought to be an increase in the relative estrogen to androgen ratio, which may occur by either increased estrogen or decreased androgen availability to breast tissue.[1,2] Androgens have an inhibitory effect on glandular development, whereas estrogens stimulate its growth. Factors that contribute to the overall estrogen/androgen environment in breast tissue include the initial production of testosterone and estrogen by the testes as well as peripheral conversion of androgens to estrogens by the enzyme *aromatase* primarily in adipose tissue.[1,2] Additionally, the serum concentration of sex hormone-binding globulin (SHBG) and the intactness of the androgen receptor pathways that lead to gene activation and transcription can alter the relative availability of estrogens and androgens under certain circumstances.[1,2]

In pubertal gynecomastia, the predominant cause of ductal hyperplasia may be related to a temporary increase in testicular production of estrogen compared with testosterone that occurs during puberty. Additionally, *aromatase* activity in peripheral tissues is thought to be higher during puberty and may increase the amount of estrogen available to breast tissue.[1] Interestingly, serum concentrations of testosterone, androstenolone, and estradiol in patients that develop pubertal gynecomastia have not been found to differ significantly when compared with patients without gynecomastia.[2] However, free testosterone (ie, testosterone not bound to SHBG or albumin) was found to be lower in these patients.[2] The cumulative effect of these processes can be described by the free hormone hypothesis. In the blood, testosterone exists in 3 major forms: free testosterone (2%), testosterone weakly bound to albumin (54%), and testosterone tightly bound to SHBG (44%).[13,14] According to the free hormone hypothesis, only free testosterone and testosterone bound to albumin are accessible to target tissues and together comprise the total bioavailable testosterone in the blood.

Additionally, the affinity of SHBG for androgen substrate is greater than that for estrogens.[1] It is likely that an increase in serum SHBG would disproportionally reduce bioavailable testosterone relative to estrogen and might explain the decrease in free testosterone levels seen in patients suffering from pubertal gynecomastia.

Most cases of pubertal gynecomastia will resolve without intervention within 18 months.[1,4] This is likely due to an equilibration of free testosterone during puberty. It is important to note that these temporary hormone fluctuations can have a lasting effect. When pubertal gynecomastia persists beyond 1 year, fibrosis of the glandular tissue can occur, which decreases the likelihood that the condition will spontaneously regress independent of treatment.[1]

Gynecomastia as a result of pharmacologic intervention may comprise upward of 10% to 25% of all reported cases.[15] Drugs strongly associated with gynecomastia including spironolactone, cimetidine, ketoconazole, human growth hormone, estrogens, human chorionic gonadotropin (hCG), antiandrogens, gonadotropin releasing hormone agonists, and 5-α reductase inhibitors.[15] Other drugs that may also be associated with gynecomastia are risperidone, verapamil, nifedipine, omeprazole, alkylating agents, efavirenz, anabolic steroids, alcohol, marijuana, and opioids.[9,15] All of these drugs are thought to either directly or indirectly affect the relative estrogen to androgen availability to breast tissue. Additionally, case reports of topical products containing lavender and tea tree oils may suggest an association of such products with the development of gynecomastia.[16]

Pathologic conditions that may cause gynecomastia include cirrhosis, malnutrition, hypogonadism (primary and secondary), Klinefelter syndrome, testicular tumors (Leydig and Sertoli cell varieties), hCG-secreting tumors, hyperthyroidism, and chronic kidney disease.[1,2] More commonly, increased adipose tissue as seen in obesity and aging may upregulate the enzyme *aromatase* and contribute to the development of gynecomastia in these populations.[1,2] It is important to keep in mind that most gynecomastia cases are idiopathic and may result from the interaction of multiple mechanisms.[2,9]

Workup and Diagnosis

The workup and diagnosis of gynecomastia can be challenging, with 25% to 58% of cases having no clear cause.[1,2,9] As with other breast masses, workup begins with a thorough history elucidating when the growth was first detected, for how long, how fast it has grown, and associated symptoms such as pain, skin changes, nipple discharge, and weight gain or loss. It is also important to conduct a complete review of systems to detect causes such as endocrine, renal, or liver pathologic condition.[17] The patient's medications and nonprescription drug use (alcohol, tobacco, marijuana, testosterone, anabolic steroids, dietary supplements, and so forth) should also be reviewed.

Physical examination is performed with the patient both in a seated, upright position and in the supine position.[18] Breast tissue should be examined in a consistent, methodical fashion using the thumb and forefinger, ensuring that all areas of the breast are palpated. It is important to note the laterality, texture of tissue, location, tenderness, and if there are any palpable lymph nodes. Gynecomastia should be bilateral, glandular (rubbery), located underneath the nipple areolar complex (NAC), nontender, and without associated discharge or palpable lymph nodes.[17,18] If the patient presents in the early, growth phase of gynecomastia they may report tenderness. Additionally, some patients may also present with unilateral or asymmetric gynecomastia.[11] In comparison, male breast cancer will commonly be unilateral and can be firm, tender, located away from the NAC, and associated with discharge or nipple retraction.[1] The remainder of the physical examination should be tailored to the patient's history, potentially consisting of a thyroid examination, assessing for liver and kidney disease, secondary sexual development, and any testicular mass or enlargement because these positive findings can help establish the cause.

Laboratory evaluation should be guided by the history and physical examination findings. Thyroid, renal, and hepatic function tests should be obtained, as should serum levels of testosterone, prolactin, follicle-stimulating hormone, and luteinizing hormone.[17,19,20] Although not a common cause of gynecomastia, hyperprolactinemia can be evaluated with serum prolactin.[21] If there is concern for malignancy-associated gynecomastia, serum levels of estrogen, hCG, dehydroepiandrosterone, and urinary 17-ketosteroids should also be obtained. Karyotype testing can also be performed if there is concern for Klinefelter syndrome.[19]

Contrary to workup of female breast masses, routine mammography and breast ultrasonography are not recommended unless there is suspicion for breast cancer or unilateral breast enlargement is present, in which case it is appropriate to perform mammography and ultrasound, and if positive, core needle biopsy (CNB).[17,22-24] If there is concern for distant tumor or malignancy as the cause, then testicular ultrasound, abdominal and/or chest computed tomography (CT) should be obtained.

Medical Treatment

Medical management of gynecomastia should be centered around physical examination, imaging/biopsy, and laboratory findings. Underlying conditions such as malignancy or endocrine disorders should be addressed first because resolution of the condition can reduce the amount of glandular tissue. Offending medications and drugs should be discontinued when possible. For idiopathic and pubertal cases, selective estrogen receptor modulator (SERM) therapy with raloxifene and tamoxifen can be effective.[18,25] SERM therapy can also be trialed in patients who have refractory gynecomastia in which the underlying cause has been treated. Aromatase inhibitor therapy can also be useful in the treatment of true gynecomastia. Anastrozole has been found to be effective in pubertal gynecomastia[18]; however, in adults it has been found to have little to no effect.[26] Testosterone has been reported to be successful in cases of hypogonadism[27]; however, it may increase gynecomastia rather than decrease the amount of tissue, particularly if the patient is eugonadal.

In situations where the offending medication cannot be discontinued, such as with androgen deprivation therapy for prostate cancer, treatment with tamoxifen or raloxifene together with radiation has been found to significantly reduce gynecomastia.[28,29]

Most cases of gynecomastia are benign and self-limiting; however, if gynecomastia has been present for greater than 12 months, it is unlikely that it will resolve with discontinuation of offending medications or with medical treatment because the glandular tissue has likely developed irreversible fibrosis and hyalinization.[17] In these scenarios, surgical excision by an experienced plastic surgeon is the most effective treatment. It is important to note that gynecomastia itself is a benign condition and does not need treatment unless there are aesthetic and psychological reasons for pursuing treatment.

Surgical Management

The most effective treatment of gynecomastia is surgery. However, as stated above, before consideration of any surgery, it is necessary that every patient has a complete medical and physical evaluation, hormone levels, review of medications and supplements, ultrasound, and ruling out any other systemic diseases.[21,30]

Surgical treatment is typically reserved for patients with long-lasting gynecomastia without spontaneous regression or refractory to medical treatment, usually after 6 months to 1 year of observation since the initial presentation in adults, and up to 2 years in pubertal patients.[30–32] Surgery is routinely performed on an outpatient basis. Several surgical techniques and combinations have been described that depend on the grade of gynecomastia.[33] The Simon classification is the most used, followed by the Rohrich classification.[32,34] The Simon classification places emphasis on the degree of enlargement and presence of excess skin, whereas the Rohrich classification places emphasis on the degree of enlargement and ptosis while also differentiating on the type of tissue present. (**Tables 1** and **2**)

Surgical procedures

The major principle of gynecomastia surgery is restoring the chest shape with minimal scar.[35] Although there are many surgical techniques described in the literature, the most commonly used technique is the skin-sparing mastectomy.[36]

Based on the Simon classification of gynecomastia, patients with grade I usually undergo liposuction, because this is very effective for the small amount of tissue present, and decreased risk of scar formation.[21] Although water-assisted and laser-assisted liposuction can be used, ultrasound-assisted liposuction (UAL) is the most recommended for its improved ability to reduce the density of fibroconnective tissue, especially when working close to the skin.[32,37,38] When performing liposuction, the ports are usually located at the lateral inframammary line with a superior pointing angle at the anterior axillary line or periareolar region.[21] Additional options for this grade of gynecomastia include the combination of liposuction and nipple sparing mastectomy (NSM) with a periareolar or inframammary incision, or the microdebrider excision and liposuction.[21,30,36,37] It is important to note that the residual subareolar glandular tissue usually causes patient dissatisfaction, which needs to be excised primarily or using a staged procedure via the liposuction incision with pull-through, or periareolar or transareolar incisions.[21,39,40] **Fig. 1** shows before and after photographs of liposuction with periareolar excision.

Simon grade IIa is usually treated depending on the size of NAC. If there is no enlargement, NSM with liposuction has demonstrated excellent outcomes. For these patients, the Pintaguy technique using a transareolar approach or Webster technique with an inferior periareolar approach are well accepted.[35] Other techniques available are the vacuum-assisted mastectomy and endoscopic mastectomy.

Another option for patients with Simon grade IIa with enlarged NAC and grade IIb is mastectomy with skin resection (MSR) via periareolar incision, or Davidson technique with liposuction, to remove the excess skin.[35] Other techniques described include the inferior deepithelialized pedicle with an inframammary incision or boomerang pattern reduction. The periareolar approach is the most recommended for patients who require skin resection because it achieves the best aesthetic acceptable outcomes.

Table 1
Simon classification[34]

Grade	Description
I	Small enlargement, no excess skin
IIa	Moderate enlargement, no excess skin
IIb	Moderate enlargement, excess skin present
III	Marked enlargement with excess skin present

Table 2
Rohrich classification[32]

Grade	Description
Grade I	Minimal hypertrophy (<250g of breast tissue) without ptosis
IA	Minimal hypertrophy—primarily glandular
IB	Minimal hypertrophy—primarily fibrous
Grade II	Moderate hypertrophy (250–500 g of breast tissue) without ptosis
IIA	Moderate hypertrophy—primarily glandular
IIB	Moderate hypertrophy—primarily fibrous
Grade III	Severe hypertrophy (>500g of breast tissue) with grade I ptosis (glandular or fibrous)
Grade IV	Severe hypertrophy with grade II or III ptosis (glandular or fibrous)

In addition, the UAL with "pull-through" excision or "orange peel" technique has shown promising results for low grades of gynecomastia, where the subareolar tissue is excised through a minimal incision with excellent results and minimal complications.[41–43] Sometimes, this method requires 2-staged procedures, with the second one in 6 to 9 months after UAL, which allows the revascularization of the NAC and due to the skin retraction in grades IIb and III, might obviate further surgeries.[41]

For patients with grade III or severe grade of gynecomastia, there are several techniques published; however, it depends on the distance from the nipple to the inframammary fold. If the distance is less than 10 cm, previously described techniques used for Simon grade IIa and IIb can be used.[36,37] However, if the distance is more than 10 cm, due to concern for pedicle perfusion, they usually undergo simple mastectomy with a free NAC graft.[21,37] Before and after pictures of simple mastectomy with free NAC graft can be seen in **Fig. 2**. For patients who desire to preservation of areolar pigmentation and nipple sensation, elliptical excision patterns may be an alternative.[21] Moreover, a new technique has been described with the preservation of NAC positioned at 16 cm from the clavicle, which consists of liposuction, MSR through an inframammary fold incision with a wide de-epithelialized postero-inferior dermal pedicle.[44,45]

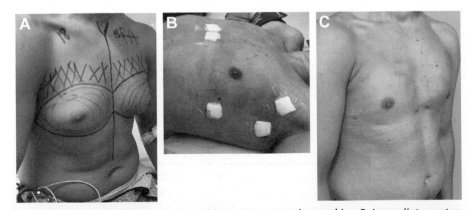

Fig. 1. Liposuction with periareolar excision. A. Preoperative marking B. Immediate postoperative appearance C. Postoperative appearance at follow-up visit.

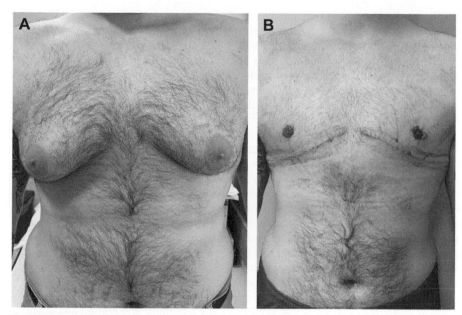

Fig. 2. Simple mastectomy with free nipple–areolar complex graft. (*A*) Preoperative marking (*B*) Postoperative appearance at follow-up visit.

In the setting of pseudogynecomastia, liposuction alone is usually preferred.[37] For all types of gynecomastia, the only contraindication for liposuction and close techniques is in patients with Klinefelter who have 50-fold to 60-fold of greater risk for breast cancer, for who mastectomy is recommended.[41] Despite an incidence of breast cancer of 1% in men, all the tissue removed should undergo histopathologic analysis.[37,44]

Outcomes and complications
The overall complication rate is 0% to 53%. This large range of complication rate is explained by the fact that different surgical approaches have different complications profiles. Hematoma is the most common presentation, with an incidence of 4.6% to 5.8%, followed by seroma in 2.4% of patients.[21,36,46,47] Late complications are usually cosmetic and due to inadequate resection of glandular tissue or skin,[21] which can typically be corrected with second-stage procedures. It is crucial to identify the difference between incomplete resection versus recurrence, which should raise the suspicion of an underlying disease, typically noted by nonfibrotic glands on pathologic condition.[21,37,48] Complications involving the NAC, such as indentation and necrosis, occur at low rates and can be avoided by leaving 2 to 10 mm of retroareolar tissue.[36] Systemic complications tend to be minimal in gynecomastia surgery.[33]

Patient-focused outcomes are typically related to aesthetics. Multiple studies have demonstrated that even in the setting of high complications, patient satisfaction can be up to 85%.[35,48]

OTHER BENIGN BREAST DISEASE
Breast Cysts

Breast cysts are fluid-filled sacs within the breast and occur very rarely in men.[49] Few cases have been reported in the literature; however, its consideration in the differential diagnosis between benign and malignant lesions in the male breast is crucial.[50] Due to anatomy, it is the most common type of breast mass in females with a lifetime prevalence of 70% to 90%; whereas in men, its incidence is very low.[50,51] Among male breast masses, cysts are usually less frequent than gynecomastia, lipomas, and epidermal inclusion cysts.[52] Their main cause is dilatation of the ducts, usually composed of ductal epithelium similar to apocrine sweat glands. Moreover, they are usually found as single lesions, associated with gynecomastia and cause alarm due to its singularity and solid consistency.[53]

Histologically, male and female breasts are different. In men, the breast usually consists of subcutaneous fat with few ducts and stroma, whereas in women, it mostly composed of ducts and glandular tissue surrounded of stroma.[2,52] Simple breast cysts occur due to the obstruction of a terminal duct from lobular hyperplasia of the epithelium or ductal extrusion into the stroma with consequent inflammation, forming an epithelium-lined fluid-filled round structure.[50,54] Gynecomastia can be associated with lobular units in male breasts, which increases the probability of cyst formation; however, cysts without gynecomastia suggest ductal origin. Maimone and colleagues found that among 5425 men who had breast imaging, 19 (0.4%) had parenchymal breast cysts, 58% of which were associated with gynecomastia.[55] Additionally, there is a proposed hypothesis of low androgen to estrogen ratio or estrogen stimulation.[52]

Breast cysts in men can be classified similarly to breast cysts in women. According to the location, they can be single, diffuse, in any quadrant, and sometimes bilateral. With regards to structure, they can be simple, complicated, or complex.[50,52] They are usually asymptomatic but can be reported as palpable, mobile, tender or nontender, and sometimes associated with nipple discharge. The frequency of clinical symptoms has been reported to be 2.4% in 2008, and imaging is usually the next step in the evaluation.[49,52,56]

The workup of breast cysts is identical to that of gynecomastia and other breast masses, consisting of clinical evaluation by a physician, imaging, and possible biopsy. Under ultrasonography, features of a simple cyst are well-defined margins, internal anechoic content, lateral acoustic shadows with posterior wall acoustic enhancement.[53] Under color-Doppler, it may have perilesional signal caused by compression of surrounding vascular structures.[53] Under mammography, they are usually seen as solitary or multiple, unilateral or bilateral, small, round, oval or lobulated, well-defined, equal or low density mass, located within the breast parenchyma.[55]

Management is similar to that of breast cysts in women. If classic benign imaging characteristics are found, there is no need for a biopsy or follow-up, and the prognosis is excellent.[52,55] However, a fine needle aspiration cytology or CNB under ultrasound guidance is warranted if any suspicious features are found as solid components seen as hypoechoic formations or vegetations, septations, noncircumscribed margins, irregular shape, thick walls, and under color Doppler it may have intralesional signals.[53,57] Despite a likelihood of malignancy of less than 2% in women, there are some case reports in male population to take in consideration when features described above are identified (56, 59–62).[55,58–61]

Lipomas

Lipomas are benign tumors of mature white fat cells contained within a fibrous capsule and are the most common neoplasm of the male breast.[62–64] Lipomas arise within the subcutaneous tissue but may occasionally extend deeper into neighboring muscle and fascia. The typical characteristic of a lipoma is a slow-growing mass with well-circumscribed margins with an overall diameter of less than 5 cm. Lipomas are rarely painful and usually represent a primarily cosmetic concern to the patient. Peak incidence of newly diagnosed lipomas is between 40 and 60 years old, although discovery of lipomas in other age groups is not uncommon. Lipomas exist as a single lesion in up to 95% of all cases but may be multiple in rare instances. Discovery of multiple lipomas in a single patient may increase the likelihood of an underlying genetic condition such as familial multiple lipomatosis or increase clinical suspicion for malignancy. The overall risk of malignant transformation of lipoma to liposarcoma is generally accepted to be approximately 1%.[63]

Most diagnoses of lipomas are made clinically by inspection and palpation alone. Findings consistent with lipomas are a well-circumscribed, subcutaneous mass that is mobile under the skin. The mass should be soft, painless, and nontender. Most commonly, lipomas exist as a singular lesion that is less than 5 cm in diameter. Patient history will often reveal that the mass has been present for a substantial amount of time and has not dramatically increased in size. Findings that increase suspicion for liposarcoma include a mass greater than 5 cm in diameter, immobilization, muscular involvement, irregular margins, multiple masses, pain, rapid growth, or a firm, nodular texture.

If physical examination findings are consistent with lipoma (ie, <5 cm), no imaging studies are indicated. However, if physical examination findings are equivocal or suspicious for malignancy (ie, >5 cm), further imaging studies should be performed.[63] Ultrasound, CT, and MRI can be used in the diagnosis, with MRI reported as the most sensitive method.[62-64] In general, histology plays little role in diagnosis unless there is significant concern for malignancy. Referral for genetic testing is only indicated when suspicion is high for an underlying genetic condition such as familial multiple lipomatosis.[63] The predominant indications for treatment include cosmetics, pain, functional impairment, or clinical findings suspicious for liposarcoma. Traditionally, management of lipomas has been limited to simple excision or liposuction. However, recent literature has highlighted the potential role for deoxycholate injections in reducing the overall volume of lipomas by approximately 75%, providing a potential future alternative to surgery. Further research into the safety and efficacy of deoxycholate injections in the treatment of lipomas is ongoing.[63-65]

The most common method for treating lipomas is surgical excision. Typically, the procedure can be performed in the office or operating room under local anesthesia. Minimal preoperative planning is required for excision of a simple lipoma. An elliptical incision should be made directly above the mass and extended to approximately two-thirds the diameter. A combination of blunt and sharp dissection should be used to fully excise the mass along with electrocautery to achieve hemostasis. Approximation of the wound is achieved via absorbable subcutaneous sutures followed by wound closure with nonabsorbable sutures. The recurrence rate for surgically excised lipomas is approximately 1% to 2%.[63] Alternative methods for the removal of lipomas include liposuction or a combination of liposuction and surgical resection. The main benefit of liposuction is a smaller, more cosmetic incision. However, controversy exists over the accuracy of histologic determinations on samples obtained from liposuction, thereby limiting the ability to rule out the possibility of liposarcoma. Additionally, the rate of recurrence for lipomas treated with liposuction is thought to be higher than for surgical excision.[63,66,67]

Pseudoangiomatous Stromal Hyperplasia

Pseudoangiomatous stromal hyperplasia (PASH) is another benign condition that can be seen in men. PASH is a proliferation of mesenchymal breast tissue, specifically stromal myofibroblasts, due to hormonal stimulation.[68] In women, PASH is a rare condition, with reports in the literature consisting of small sample size case reports.[69]

Given the link to hormonal stimulation, it is a very rare condition to see in men and can often be linked to gynecomastia.[68,70–72] Although benign, it is important to distinguish this condition from low-grade angiosarcoma.[68] Workup of this condition begins with a thorough history and physical examination, looking for distinguishing findings such as tenderness, texture, size, mobile versus fixed, and location. Radiographic workup begins with mammography, in which PASH seems as an oval mass without microcalcifications.[70,71] Ultrasound can then be used to further assess the mass, with the distinguishing finding of a hypoechoic mass.[56] Definitive diagnosis is made with tissue biopsy, with the gold standard being CNB.[70] On biopsy, the characteristic findings are slit-like spaces lined by myofibroblasts, which resemble vascular spaces (leading to the pseudoangiomatous name), as well as a collagen-based stroma.[68,70] Immunohistochemistry can be used to differentiate from low-grade angiosarcoma because the sample will stain in the profile of myofibroblasts.[70]

Management of this condition frequently consists of surgical excision.[68] However, given the extremely low potential for malignant transformation, it is reasonable to consider observation after discussion at tumor board with serial mammography if core biopsy is confirmatory for PASH and there is a negative family history of breast cancer.[69,71] It is also reasonable to pursue surgical excision for cosmetic reasons should the appearance of a breast mass be bothersome given the low amount of baseline breast tissue in men. Regardless of the indication, surgical excision should proceed as a standard breast surgical biopsy, involving a needle-guided excision.

Breast Infections

Infections of the breast are yet another condition that can affect men. Types of infections can include cellulitis, breast abscess, and skin abscess overlying the breast. Cellulitis will present as pain, erythema, tenderness, and warmth. Risk factors for cellulitis include prior infection, recent surgery, trauma, or lesions such as eczema.[73–75] The most common pathogens are beta-hemolytic streptococci.[74,75] Diagnosis consists of thorough history and physical examination, ruling out any suspicious masses or fluid collections.[76] If there is suspicion for abscess or mass, imaging can be obtained using ultrasound and mammography.[77,78] If cellulitis is confirmed, treatment should consist of antibiotics to cover common skin flora–specific regimens are covered in this section on antibiotics. Anti-inflammatory medications such as ibuprofen can be used to reduce pain and discomfort.

Skin abscesses can result from epidermoid cysts and hidradenitis suppurativa. The most common pathogens are *Staphylococcus aureus* and beta-hemolytic streptococci.[79] As previously described, workup should consist of a thorough history and physical examination, with imaging obtained as needed. Incision and drainage should be performed, as described in this section on incision and drainage. A culture should be obtained, and the patient should be started on antibiotics, as described below. The patient should receive close follow-up to ensure resolution.

Breast abscesses can occur as a primary process, or commonly as a complication of mastitis.[80] Primary breast abscesses are associated with many risk factors such as diabetes mellitus, obesity, and tobacco smoking.[81] Fundamentally, there should be some explanation for why an abscess has occurred, which also includes breast cancer in the differential and a thorough history and physical examination with appropriate imaging should rule out breast cancer as a possible cause especially in patients with personal or family risk factors for breast cancer. A breast abscess is most commonly due to *S. aureus* infection.[81] Patients can frequently present with fever and malaise, and a painful, fluctuant mass. If the overlying skin seems normal, needle aspiration under ultrasound guidance can be used to drain the cavity and obtain a culture to guide antibiotic therapy.[82] If needle aspiration is performed, close follow-up is needed to monitor for resolution of the abscess, which is defined as an abscess cavity without pus, or with serous fluid.[80] Repeat aspirations may be needed for resolution. If there is evidence of skin ischemia or necrosis, or if the abscess does not improve with needle aspiration, incision and drainage can be performed.[83] This can be performed as described below. Following drainage and culture, the patient should be started on antibiotics and seen in follow-up to ensure resolution.

An incision and drainage of the breast can be performed as follows. The skin should be prepped with antiseptic solution, and the area should be infiltrated with local anesthetic. A linear incision should be made, taking care to follow Langer's lines to improve final cosmetic appearance. A culture should be taken, and then the fluid should be drained out. If there is clinical suspicion, a small breast specimen could be obtained and sent to pathology to rule out breast cancer. Once drained, a probe should be used to determine if there are any loculated areas.[84] Once completely drained, the cavity should be irrigated with saline.[85] Then, it should be allowed it to heal by secondary intention with packing/dressing changes. If the abscess is large, or the patient is immunocompromised or diabetic, packing should be used to prevent recurrence.

Antibiotic choice should be tailored to the patient's clinical condition. Oral antibiotic regimens are often appropriate; however, intravenous antibiotics should be used if the patient has signs of systemic infection. Antibiotic therapy should provide coverage for *S. aureus* and is tailored to the culture data.[81] The first-line oral antibiotics include cephalexin, clindamycin, and trimethoprim sulfamethoxazole, typically administered for a 10-day to 14-day course.[81,86] For more severe infections requiring hospitalization, appropriate intravenous choices include ampicillin-sulbactam, or vancomycin if there is concern for methicillin resistant *S. aureus* infection.

Seromas

A seroma is a subcutaneous collection of fluid comprising a mixture of plasma, lymph, and inflammatory exudate and is a common complication associated with many surgical procedures.[87,88] The pathophysiologic mechanism underlying seroma formation is likely related to transection of lymphatics during the surgical procedure resulting in leakage of lymph and production of an inflammatory exudate by the damaged tissue.[89,90] Surgical procedures that involve the creation of anatomic dead space have an increased likelihood of developing seromas. Surgical techniques that increase inflammation, such as the use of electrocautery or prophylactic sclerosants, are also associated with increased risk of seromas, as is early postoperative mobilization.[87,91,92] Overall, seromas represent a common cause of patient discomfort during the postoperative period and often require drainage to prevent infection. In rare instances, reoperation may be necessary.[87]

The diagnosis of a postoperative complication of seroma is most often a clinical diagnosis. On physical examination, a seroma should seem as a subcutaneous bulge with a positive fluid wave. Signs of inflammation may or may not be present. Seromas are typically not painful, although patients may indicate the presence of an uncomfortable sensation or pressure under the skin. Finally, ultrasound is a sensitive and cost-effective method that is routinely used to assist in the workup and diagnosis.[93]

In general, most symptomatic seromas should be treated with needle aspiration using sterile technique under local anesthesia and wrapped in a compression bandage. Occasionally, repeated drainage may be necessary. Small, asymptomatic seromas tend to resolve spontaneously and may not require drainage.[94]

Importantly, evidence-based strategies for the prevention of postoperative seroma formation should be used by all practicing surgeons during the initial surgery. Efforts should be made during the index procedure to minimize dead space, shear stress, and electrocautery to help reduce the risk of seromas. Furthermore, the use of drains postoperative has also been associated with a reduced risk of seroma formation.[87]

CLINICS CARE POINTS

- Gynecomastia is the benign proliferation of glandular breast tissue.
- Gynecomastia can be seen in men of all ages; however, most frequently occurs in neonates, adolescents, and older men.
- Most cases of adolescent gynecomastia will spontaneously resolve within 1 year.
- Gynecomastia in adults is often secondary to medication, alcohol, or marijuana use. Cessation of the offending agent(s) may improve the condition.
- Laboratory tests useful in the workup of gynecomastia include the following:
  - Thyroid-stimulating hormone
  - Triiodothyronine
  - Alanine transaminase
  - Alkaline phosphatase
  - Creatinine
  - Testosterone
  - Prolactin
  - Follicle-stimulating hormone
  - Luteinizing hormone
- Gynecomastia lasting longer than 1 year typically requires medical or surgical intervention for resolution to occur.
- Medical management of gynecomastia may include tamoxifen (first-line), other SERMs (raloxifene and clomiphene), and aromatase inhibitor s (anastrozole and testolactone). Early initiation of therapy increases the likelihood for successful treatment.
- Surgery is a safe and effective treatment of gynecomastia and should be considered in cases that persist longer than 1 year or are refractory to medical management.
- Breast cysts in men are rare; however, it can be associated with gynecomastia.
- The workup of male breast cysts should involve thorough history and physical examination, as well as imaging and possible biopsy to rule out malignancy.
- Management of breast cysts in men depends on imaging and biopsy findings and can vary from watchful waiting to surgical excision.
- Lipomas are the most common benign breast neoplasms in men, consisting of mature fat cells contained in a fibrous capsule, usually found in the subcutaneous plane.
- Diagnosis is made through history, inspection, and palpation, demonstrated a long standing, slow growing, mobile mass often measuring less than 5 cm.
- Unless there are concerning features of malignancy, lipomas are often only excised for cosmetic reasons or for patient comfort.
- Pseudoangiomatous stromal hyperplasia (PASH) is a rare condition in men, consisting of abnormal proliferation of mesenchymal breast tissue that can resemble angiosarcoma.
- PASH is often diagnosed through imaging or biopsy and can be found during pathologic examination of gynecomastia specimens.
- PASH may be excised using a surgical biopsy if patient is concerned but it is a benign process, and watchful waiting can be used in the appropriate patient.
- Breast infections are another common benign breast lesion in men, most frequently consisting of cellulitis, skin abscess, or primary breast abscess.

- Workup of breast infections should be performed to rule out malignancy.
- The mainstay of treatment of breast infections includes antibiotics treatment, and in the case of abscesses, aspiration or surgical drainage.
- Seromas can be seen in male patients following surgical procedures on or near the breast and are often related to the disruption of lymphatics and local inflammation.
- Seromas are often diagnosed through physical examination and ultrasonography.
- Management of seromas involves aspiration of the fluid collection followed by compression of the site.

DISCLOSURE

The authors have nothing to disclose.

REFERENCES

1. Braunstein GD. Clinical practice. Gynecomastia. N Engl J Med 2007;357(12): 1229–37.
2. Johnson RE, Murad MH. Gynecomastia: pathophysiology, evaluation, and management. Mayo Clin Proc 2009;84(11):1010–5.
3. Mathur R, Braunstein GD. Gynecomastia: pathomechanisms and treatment strategies. Horm Res 1997;48(3):95–102.
4. Kanakis GA, Nordkap L, Bang AK, et al. EAA clinical practice guidelines-gynecomastia evaluation and management. Andrology 2019;7(6):778–93.
5. Nydick M, Bustos J, Dale JH Jr, et al. Gynecomastia in adolescent boys. JAMA 1961;178:449–54.
6. Moore DC, Schlaepfer LV, Paunier L, et al. Hormonal changes during puberty: V. Transient pubertal gynecomastia: abnormal androgen-estrogen ratios. J Clin Endocrinol Metab 1984;58(3):492–9.
7. Biro FM, Lucky AW, Huster GA, et al. Hormonal studies and physical maturation in adolescent gynecomastia. J Pediatr 1990;116(3):450–5. https://doi.org/10.1016/s0022-3476(05)82843-4.
8. Braunstein GD. What Accounts for the Increased Incidence of Gynecomastia Diagnosis in Denmark from 1998–2017? J Clin Endocrinol Metab 2020;105(10): e3810–1.
9. Mieritz MG, Christiansen P, Jensen MB, et al. Gynaecomastia in 786 adult men: clinical and biochemical findings. Eur J Endocrinol 2017;176(5):555–66.
10. Nuttall FQ. Gynecomastia as a physical finding in normal men. J Clin Endocrinol Metab 1979;48(2):338–40.
11. Niewoehner CB, Nuttal FQ. Gynecomastia in a hospitalized male population. Am J Med 1984;77(4):633–8.
12. Georgiadis E, Papandreou L, Evangelopoulou C, et al. Incidence of gynaecomastia in 954 young males and its relationship to somatometric parameters. Ann Hum Biol 1994;21(6):579–87.
13. DUNN JF, NISULA BC, RODBARD D. Transport of steroid hormones: binding of 21 endogenous steroids to both testosterone-binding globulin and corticosteroid-binding globulin in human plasma. J Clin Endocrinol Metab 1981;53(1):58–68.
14. Vermeulen A. Physiology of the testosterone-binding globulin in man. Ann N Y Acad Sci 1988;538:103–11.

15. Deepinder F, Braunstein GD. Drug-induced gynecomastia: an evidence-based review. Expert Opin Drug Saf 2012;11(5):779–95.

16. Ramsey JT, Li Y, Arao Y, et al. Lavender products associated with premature thelarche and prepubertal gynecomastia: case reports and endocrine-disrupting chemical activities. J Clin Endocrinol Metab 2019;104(11):5393–405.

17. Malata CM and Wong KY. Gynecomastia Surgery. In: Nahabedian MY and Neligan PC. Plastic Surgery.

18. Fitzgerald PA. Gynecomastia. In: Papadakis MA, McPhee SJ, Rabow MW, et al, editors. Current medical diagnosis & treatment. 2022.

19. Sansone A, Romanelli F, Sansone M, et al. Gynecomastia and hormones. Endocrine 2017;55(1):37–44. Epub 2016 May 4. PMID: 27145756.

20. Dickson G. Gynecomastia. Am Fam Physician 2012;85(7):716–22. PMID: 22534349.

21. Brown RH, Chang DK, Siy R, et al. Trends in the surgical correction of gynecomastia. Semin Plast Surg 2015;29(2):122–30.

22. Muñoz Carrasco R, Alvarez Benito M, Muñoz Gomariz E, et al. Mammography and ultrasound in the evaluation of male breast disease. Eur Radiol 2010; 20(12):2797–805. Epub 2010 Jun 23. PMID: 20571799.

23. Westenend PJ. Core needle biopsy in male breast lesions. J Clin Pathol 2003; 56(11):863–5. PMID: 14600134; PMCID: PMC1770095.

24. Janes SE, Lengyel JA, Singh S, et al. Needle core biopsy for the assessment of unilateral breast masses in men. Breast 2006;15(2):273–5. Epub 2005 Jul 18. PMID: 16026984.

25. Lawrence SE, Faught KA, Vethamuthu J, et al. Beneficial effects of raloxifene and tamoxifen in the treatment of pubertal gynecomastia. J Pediatr 2004;145(1):71–6. PMID: 15238910.

26. Chapter 384: Disorders of the Testes and Male Reproductive System. In: Jameson JL, Fauci AS, Kasper DL, Hauser SL, Longo DL, Loscalzo J. Harrison's Principles of Internal Medicine. 20th edition.

27. Gruntmanis U, Braunstein GD. Treatment of gynecomastia. Curr Opin Investig Drugs 2001;2(5):643–9. PMID: 11569940.

28. Baumgarten L, Dabaja AA. Diagnosis and management of gynecomastia for urologists. Curr Urol Rep 2018;19(7):46. PMID: 29774423.

29. Nguyen PL, Alibhai SM, Basaria S, et al. Adverse effects of androgen deprivation therapy and strategies to mitigate them. Eur Urol 2015;67(5):825–36. Epub 2014 Aug 2. PMID: 25097095.

30. Schröder L, Rudlowski C, Walgenbach-Brünagel G, et al. Surgical strategies in the treatment of gynecomastia grade I-II: the combination of liposuction and subcutaneous mastectomy provides excellent patient outcome and satisfaction. Breast care (Basel, Switzerland) 2015;10(3):184–8.

31. Kanakis GA, Nordkap L. EAA Clin Pract guidelines-gynecomastia Eval Manag 2019;7(6):778–93.

32. Rohrich RJ, Ha RY, Kenkel JM, et al. Classification and management of gynecomastia: defining the role of ultrasound-assisted liposuction. Plast Reconstr Surg 2003;111(2):909–23 ; discussion 24-5.

33. Zavlin D, Jubbal KT, Friedman JD, et al. Complications and outcomes after gynecomastia surgery: analysis of 204 pediatric and 1583 adult cases from a national multi-center database. Aesthetic Plast Surg 2017;41(4):761–7.

34. Simon BE, Hoffman S, Kahn S. Classification and surgical correction of gynecomastia. Plast Reconstr Surg 1973;51(1):48–52.

35. Longheu A, Medas F, Corrias F, et al. Surgical management of gynecomastia: experience of a general surgery center. Il Giornale di chirurgia 2016;37(4):150–4.
36. Holzmer SW, Lewis PG, Landau MJ, et al. Surgical management of gynecomastia: a comprehensive review of the literature. Plast Reconstr Surg Glob open 2020;8(10):e3161–.
37. Mett TR, Pfeiler PP, Luketina R, et al. Surgical treatment of gynaecomastia: a standard of care in plastic surgery. Eur J Plast Surg 2020;43(4):389–98.
38. de Souza Pinto EB, Chiarello de Souza Pinto Abdala P, Montecinos Maciel C, et al. Liposuction and VASER. Clin Plast Surg 2006;33(1):107–15.
39. Webster JP. Mastectomy for Gynecomastia Through a Semicircular Intra-areolar Incision. Ann Surg 1946;124(3):557–75.
40. Morselli PG. Pull-through": a new technique for breast reduction in gynecomastia. Plast Reconstr Surg 1996;97(2):450–4.
41. Bailey SH, Guenther D, Constantine F, et al. Gynecomastia Management: An Evolution and Refinement in Technique at UT Southwestern Medical Center. Plast Reconstr Surg Glob open 2016;4(6):e734.
42. Shirol SS. Orange Peel excision of gland: a novel surgical technique for treatment of gynecomastia. Ann Plast Surg 2016;77(6):615–9.
43. Thiénot S, Bertheuil N, Carloni R, et al. Postero-inferior pedicle surgical technique for the treatment of grade iii gynecomastia. Aesthetic Plast Surg 2017;41(3): 531–41.
44. Fentiman IS, Fourquet A, Hortobagyi GN. Male breast cancer. Lancet (London, England) 2006;367(9510):595–604.
45. Lapid O, Jolink F. Surgical management of gynecomastia: 20 years' experience. Scand J Surg 2013;103(1):41–5.
46. Steele SR, Martin MJ, Place RJ. Gynecomastia: complications of the subcutaneous mastectomy. Am surgeon 2002;68(2):210–3.
47. Fricke A, Lehner GM, Stark GB, et al. Gynecomastia: histological appearance in different age groups. J Plast Surg Hand Surg 2018;52(3):166–71.
48. Colombo-Benkmann M, Buse B, Stern J, et al. Indications for and results of surgical therapy for male gynecomastia. Am J Surg 1999;178(1):60–3.
49. Azimi N, Azar A, Khan A, et al. Benign breast cyst in a young male. Cureus 2019; 11(6):e4814–.
50. Salemis NS. Benign cyst of the male breast. An exceedingly rare entity that may pose a diagnostic dilemma. Management and literature review. Breast Dis 2021; 40(3):207–11.
51. Kowalski A, Okoye E. StatPearls Publishing;. In: Breast cyst. [Updated 2021 Dec 13]. Treasure Island (FL): StatPearls [Internet]; 2022. Available at: https://www.ncbi.nlm.nih.gov/books/NBK562196/.
52. Parsian S, Rahbar H, Rendi MH, et al. Benign breast cyst without associated gynecomastia in a male patient: a case report. J Radiol Case Rep 2011;5(11): 35–40.
53. Draghi F, Tarantino CC, Madonia L, et al. Ultrasonography of the male breast. J Ultrasound 2011;14(3):122–9.
54. Berg WA, Sechtin AG, Marques H, et al. Cystic breast masses and the ACRIN 6666 experience. Radiol Clin North Am 2010;48(5):931–87.
55. Maimone S, Ocal IT, Robinson KA, et al. Characteristics and Management of Male Breast Parenchymal Cysts. J Breast Imaging 2020;2(4):330–5.
56. Iuanow E, Kettler M, Slanetz PJ. Spectrum of Disease in the Male Breast. Am J Roentgenol 2011;196(3):W247–59.

57. D'Orsi CJ, Sickles EA, Mendelson EB, et al. ACR BI-RADS®Atlas, breast imaging reporting and data system. Reston, VA: American College of Radiology; 2013.
58. Kinoshita H, Kashiwagi S, Teraoka H, et al. Intracystic papillary carcinoma of the male breast: a case report. World J Surg Oncol 2018;16(1):15.
59. Tochika N, Takano A, Yoshimoto T, et al. Intracystic carcinoma of the male breast: report of a case. Surg Today 2001;31(9):806–9.
60. Sinha S, Hughes RG, Ryley NG. Papillary carcinoma in a male breast cyst: a diagnostic challenge. Ann R Coll Surg Engl 2006;88(5):W3–5.
61. Ravichandran D, Carty NJ, al-Talib RK, et al. Cystic carcinoma of the breast: a trap for the unwary. Ann R Coll Surg Engl 1995;77(2):123–6.
62. Chau A, Jafarian N, Rosa M. Male breast: clinical and imaging evaluations of benign and malignant entities with histologic correlation. Am J Med 2016; 129(8):776–91.
63. Pandya KA, Radke F. Benign skin lesions: lipomas, epidermal inclusion cysts, muscle and nerve biopsies. Surg Clin North Am Jun 2009;89(3):677–87.
64. Ingraffea A. Benign skin neoplasms. Facial Plast Surg Clin North Am 2013;21(1): 21–32.
65. Amber KT, Ovadia S, Camacho I. Injection therapy for the management of superficial subcutaneous lipomas. J Clin Aesthet Dermatol 2014;7(6):46–8.
66. Gaucher S, Maladry D, Silitra AM, et al. Removal of subcutaneous lipomas: Interest of liposuction. J Cosmet Dermatol 2017;16(3):400–1.
67. Copeland-Halperin LR, Pimpinella V, Copeland M. Combined liposuction and excision of lipomas: long-term evaluation of a large sample of patients. Plast Surg Int 2015;2015:625396.
68. Maciolek LM, Harmon TS, He J, et al. Pseudoangiomatous stromal hyperplasia of the breast: a rare finding in a male patient. Cureus 2019;11(6):e4923. Published 2019 Jun 17.
69. Bowman E, Oprea G, Okoli J, et al. Pseudoangiomatous stromal hyperplasia (PASH) of the breast: a series of 24 patients. Breast J 2012;18(3):242–7.
70. Jaunoo SS, Thrush S, Dunn P. Pseudoangiomatous stromal hyperplasia (PASH): a brief review. Int J Surg 2011;9(1):20–2.
71. AlSharif S, Alshamrani KM, Scaranelo A, et al. Unusual Male Breast Lesions. J Clin Imaging Sci 2021;11:21. Published 2021 Apr 19.
72. Lattin GE Jr, Jesinger RA, Mattu R, et al. From the radiologic pathology archives: diseases of the male breast: radiologic-pathologic correlation. Radiographics 2013;33(2):461–89. https://doi.org/10.1148/rg.332125208.
73. Hughes LL, Styblo TM, Thoms WW, et al. Cellulitis of the breast as a complication of breast-conserving surgery and irradiation. Am J Clin Oncol 1997;20(4):338–41.
74. Mertz KR, Baddour LM, Bell JL, et al. Breast cellulitis following breast conservation therapy: a novel complication of medical progress. Clin Infect Dis 1998;26(2): 481–6.
75. Rescigno J, McCormick B, Brown AE, et al. Breast cellulitis after conservative surgery and radiotherapy. Int J Radiat Oncol Biol Phys 1994;29(1):163–8.
76. Zippel D, Siegelmann-Danieli N, Ayalon S, et al. Delayed breast cellulitis following breast conserving operation. Eur J Surg Oncol 2003;29(4):327–30.
77. Peters F, Petersen EE, Kirkpatrick CJ. Isolated erythema (cellulitis) of the breast. Breast 2002;11(6):484–8.
78. Rahmouni A, Chosidow O, Mathieu D, et al. MR imaging in acute infectious cellulitis. Radiology 1994;192(2):493–6.
79. Miller LG, Quan C, Shay A, et al. A prospective investigation of outcomes after hospital discharge for endemic, community-acquired methicillin-resistant and

-susceptible Staphylococcus aureus skin infection. Clin Infect Dis 2007;44(4): 483–92.

80. Dixon JM, Khan LR. Treatment of breast infection. BMJ 2011;342:d396. Published 2011 Feb 11.

81. Bharat A, Gao F, Aft RL, et al. Predictors of primary breast abscesses and recurrence. World J Surg 2009;33(12):2582–6.

82. Dixon JM. Breast abscess. Br J Hosp Med (Lond) 2007;68(6):315–20.

83. Christensen AF, Al-Suliman N, Nielsen KR, et al. Ultrasound-guided drainage of breast abscesses: results in 151 patients. Br J Radiol 2005;78(927):186–8.

84. Fitch MT, Manthey DE, McGinnis HD, et al. Videos in clinical medicine. abscess incision and drainage. N Engl J Med 2007;357(19):e20.

85. Korownyk C, Allan GM. Evidence-based approach to abscess management. Can Fam Physician 2007;53(10):1680–4.

86. Leach RD, Eykyn SJ, Phillips I, et al. Anaerobic subareolar breast abscess. Lancet 1979;1(8106):35–7.

87. Janis JE, Khansa L, Khansa I. Strategies for postoperative seroma prevention: a systematic review. Plast Reconstr Surg 2016;138(1):240–52.

88. Marangi GF, Segreto F, Morelli Coppola M, et al. Management of chronic seromas: a novel surgical approach with the use of vacuum assisted closure therapy. Int Wound J 2020;17(5):1153–8.

89. Tadych K, Donegan WL. Postmastectomy seromas and wound drainage. Surg Gynecol Obstet 1987;165(6):483–7.

90. Andrades P, Prado A, Danilla S, et al. Progressive tension sutures in the prevention of postabdominoplasty seroma: a prospective, randomized, double-blind clinical trial. Plast Reconstr Surg 2007;120(4):935–46.

91. Shamley DR, Barker K, Simonite V, et al. Delayed versus immediate exercises following surgery for breast cancer: a systematic review. Breast Cancer Res Treat 2005;90(3):263–71.

92. Yilmaz KB, Dogan L, Nalbant H, et al. Comparing scalpel, electrocautery and ultrasonic dissector effects: the impact on wound complications and pro-inflammatory cytokine levels in wound fluid from mastectomy patients. J Breast Cancer 2011;14(1):58–63.

93. Di Martino M, Nahas FX, Barbosa MVJ, et al. Seroma in lipoabdominoplasty and abdominoplasty: a comparative study using ultrasound. Plast Reconstr Surg 2010;126(5):1742–51. https://doi.org/10.1097/PRS.0b013e3181efa6c5.

94. Vidal P, Berner JE, Will PA. Managing complications in abdominoplasty: a literature review. Arch Plast Surg 2017;44(5):457–68.

Benign Breast Disease
Periareolar Mastitis, Granulomatous Lobular Mastitis, and Lymphocytic or Diabetic Mastopathy

Rachel E. Sargent, MD[a,b], Stephen F. Sener, MD, FSSO[a,b],*

KEYWORDS

- Periareolar mastitis • Granulomatous lobular mastitis • Diabetic mastopathy

KEY POINTS

- The operative management of periareolar mastitis consists of central duct excision, excision of the site of the abscess at the periareolar margin, and reconstruction of the subareolar complex.
- The authors' current treatment strategy for granulomatous lobular mastitis avoids surgical procedures in favor of aspiration of abscesses, management with short courses of antibiotics, and even observation for the treatment of milder cases of granulomatous mastitis.
- Diabetic mastopathy occurs in patients with long-standing insulin-dependent diabetes, especially those with microvascular complications such as retinopathy, nephropathy, or neuropathy. If the diagnosis can be confirmed by core needle biopsy, surgical excision can generally be avoided.

INTRODUCTION

Although the surgical treatment of *malignant* diseases of the breast is an important component of patient outcome, there are times when the technical elements of procedures for *benign* inflammatory breast conditions are underappreciated, clinically vexing, and can lead to significant morbidity when underperformed; this is certainly true for periareolar mastitis, granulomatous lobular mastitis, and lymphocytic or diabetic mastopathy, where understanding the pathophysiology is a key to success in the surgical management of these conditions.

---

[a] Department of Surgery, Los Angeles County + University of Southern California (LAC+USC) Medical Center, Los Angeles, CA, USA; [b] Department of Surgery, Keck School of Medicine of USC, University of Southern California, Los Angeles, CA, USA
* Corresponding author. Los Angeles County, 1100 North State Street, Clinic Tower, 6A231A, Los Angeles, CA 90033.
E-mail addresses: stephen.sener@med.usc.edu; sfsener@aol.com

Surg Clin N Am 102 (2022) 1007–1016
https://doi.org/10.1016/j.suc.2022.06.004
0039-6109/22/© 2022 Elsevier Inc. All rights reserved.
surgical.theclinics.com

PERIAREOLAR MASTITIS

Periareolar mastitis is also known by its synonyms periductal, subareolar, and plasma cell mastitis. It is an uncommon benign inflammatory condition of the breast that causes frustration for many patients, and its pathophysiology is misunderstood by many surgeons. Seminal clinical observations regarding diagnosis and surgical management have been provided by some of the leaders of breast surgery from previous generations, including Urban,[1] Scanlon,[2] and more recently Lannin.[3]

Clinical Presentation and Initial Treatment

Periareolar mastitis frequently presents as a recurrent abscess or sinus at the areolar margin in women in their 20s and 30s (**Fig. 1**). Although the disease process can occur in men, it is exceedingly uncommon in our experience. It is not unusual to see patients who have had either a previous incision and drainage of abscess without accompanying definitive surgical treatment or a prior breast biopsy revealing duct ectasia. Duct ectasia is a manifestation of chronic duct obstruction and is a nonspecific finding that may be associated with multiple etiologies.

The pathognomonic findings on clinical examination are erythema and edema involving the periareolar margin and a transverse cleft in the nipple itself. At times, there is enough edema in the areolar skin that the transverse cleft is not identifiable at the time of presentation, only being appreciated when the edema and erythema have somewhat resolved after initial treatment with antibiotics or drainage of an

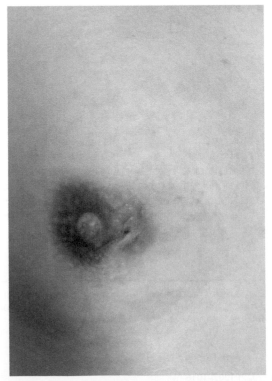

Fig. 1. Periareolar mastitis. Patient presented with 2-year history of exacerbations and remissions of inflammation at the periareolar margin, now with a chronic lactiferous sinus.

abscess. Imaging with ultrasound is preferred and demonstrates a mass within the central duct with postobstructive duct ectasia in the subareolar duct system.

Initial treatment usually consists of a short course of antibiotics and aspiration of abscess to reduce the inflammation enough so that a definitive surgical procedure can be done. Persistent or recurrent abscess may occasionally require incision and drainage, which, if necessary, should be done using only a periareolar incision to facilitate the reconstruction of the subsequent surgical defect incurred during the definitive surgical excision.

Pathophysiology and Surgical Management

The hallmark pathologic finding is squamous metaplasia of the epithelial lining of the central duct within the nipple causing major duct obstruction and subareolar duct ectasia.[4] An association between cigarette smoking and the development of squamous metaplasia has previously been described.[5] The mechanical obstruction of the central duct causes dilatation of the subareolar ducts and sets up a vicious cycle of periductal inflammatory response, infection, and further duct obstruction. However, it is not known what percentage of women with a transverse cleft in the nipple never develop a clinical infection. Antibiotics, aspiration, and incision and drainage of abscess do not address the cause of the central duct obstruction, so it is not surprising that these therapeutic maneuvers in the absence of central duct excision are associated with a disease process characterized by exacerbations and recurrence of abscess. If the condition becomes chronic, there is occasionally a periductal infiltration of plasma cells, leading to the so-called plasma cell mastitis. It is also appreciated that not all patients who have initial treatment with antibiotics and aspiration of abscess develop a recurrence of periareolar mastitis requiring central duct excision. Indeed, Lannin reported that only about one-half of patients developed a recurrent abscess after management of the first episode with antibiotics and aspiration of abscess.[3]

Indications for surgical management include persistent lactiferous duct fistula, recurrent subareolar abscess, or a residual mass remaining after needle aspiration and antibiotics. The operative management consists of central duct excision, excision of the site of the abscess at the periareolar margin, and reconstruction of the subareolar complex. Urban[1] described a radial incision, and Lannin[3] favored removing an ellipse of skin in a radial fashion. Scanlon[6] popularized the concept of "diamond biopsy," in which the central major duct, a portion of the skin of the areola and breast including the site of the abscess, and subareolar complex are excised (Fig. 2). The reconstructed nipple-areolar complex retains a reasonably natural appearance (Edward F. Scanlon, MD, 1977–1982, Evanston Hospital, Evanston, ILL, personal communications) (Fig. 3). We continue to use the "diamond biopsy" in current-day practice.

Recurrence of periareolar mastitis after definitive duct excision is highly unusual. Interesting enough, in our experience and confirmed by Lannin,[3] the development of periareolar mastitis in the contralateral breast is also uncommon.

GRANULOMATOUS LOBULAR MASTITIS

Granulomatous lobular mastitis (GLM) is an uncommon but challenging group of benign inflammatory diseases of the breast, requiring careful management of provider and patient expectations.

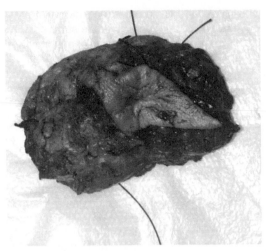

Fig. 2. "Diamond biopsy" includes excision of the central duct, the site of the abscess at the periareolar margin, and subareolar complex.

Clinical Presentation and Initial Evaluation

There have been many publications on GLM from Turkey, and in the United States greater than 90% of patients identify ethnically as Hispanic, leading some investigators to suggest that GLM has a Mediterranean origin. Patients most commonly present with a palpable breast mass at a median age of 35 years and with a recent history of pregnancy.[6] As GLM becomes a chronic condition, there is a characteristic discoloration of the skin overlying the breast mass.

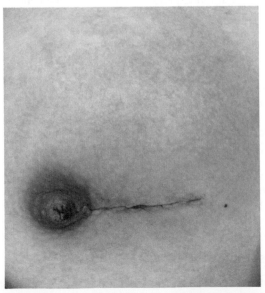

Fig. 3. Reconstructed nipple-areolar complex after excision of the central duct, skin with periareolar abscess, and subareolar complex.

Imaging should include breast ultrasound, which typically demonstrates a hypoe-choic mass with features similar to those seen in carcinoma of the breast, so core nee-dle biopsy is essential to distinguish the difference between GLM and cancer. The hallmark pathologic finding of GLM is the presence of noncaseating granulomas centered around breast lobules. Acid-fast bacillus and Grocott methenamine silver stains exclude tuberculosis and fungi as causes of GLM. A thorough review of the pa-tient's history and physical examination should be done to exclude other diseases associated with breast granulomas, such as histoplasmosis, sarcoidosis, foreign body reaction, and collagen vascular diseases (Sjogren syndrome and erythema nodosum).

Treatment of Granulomatous Lobular Mastitis and Idiopathic Granulomatous Mastitis

Cases of GLM with identifiable causes have defined treatment criteria, but those without identifiable causes are generally referred to as idiopathic granulomatous mastitis (IGM). Most patients presenting with GLM will be designated as having IGM, as demonstrated in a recent report of GLM in which only 4% of patients had co-existing autoimmune diseases.[6] Despite having been first described by Kessler and Wolloch[7] in 1972, the lack of consensus on the cause of IGM has led to multiple treatment options, ranging from observation to medical treatment with steroids, bromocriptine, methotrexate, and antibiotics to aspiration of fluid collections to surgi-cal interventions, such as incision and drainage, excision, and even mastectomy.[8-15]

In our experience treating 285 patients with GLM from 2008 to 2018 at a large urban safety-net medical center, the treatment algorithm evolved over the 10-year period.[6] Because of unfavorable cosmetic outcomes with surgical management in our early experience, the preferred treatment of fluid collections and abscesses became aspi-ration instead of incision and drainage. Fine-needle aspiration can be performed by the surgeon at the bedside with or without ultrasound guidance. Also, the use of ste-roids became reserved for patients with diseases for which steroids were the appro-priate initial management instead of being used more liberally for patients with large areas of breast involved with IGM, refractory to 4 to 6 weeks of antibiotic therapy.

For the patients in this series, once the diagnosis of IGM was confirmed by core nee-dle biopsy, 17% of patients had no treatment, 22% had aspiration (± medical treat-ment, defined as a short course of antibiotics consisting of oral trimethoprim/sulfamethoxazole and metronidazole, and nasal mupirocin), 35% had medical treat-ment alone, and 27% had surgical intervention (± medical treatment). The overall me-dian duration of disease was 16 weeks, and for patients treated by aspiration (± medical treatment) or medical treatment alone it was not significantly different than for those who were observed without treatment. However, disease duration was significantly longer for patients who had surgical intervention (± medical treatment) than for those who were observed. Patients requiring surgical intervention probably had more severe cases of IGM than those in the other treatment groups, resulting in more protracted courses of disease. The overall recurrence rate was 22%. Compared with patients who were observed, the recurrence rate was not significantly higher for patients who had aspiration (± medical treatment) or for those who received medical treatment alone, but it was significantly higher for patients who had surgical interven-tion (± medical treatment). The findings of this study appeared to justify our current treatment strategy of avoiding surgical procedures in favor of aspiration of abscesses, management with short courses of antibiotics, and even observation for the treatment of milder cases of IGM. However, one of the more difficult problems associated with this treatment algorithm was managing the understandable frustration of patients and providers during multiple recurrences of erythema and abscess, while resisting the temptation to use incision and drainage procedures.

Identifying the cause of IGM has remained elusive. It has been appreciated more recently that the microbiome can make significant contributions to granulomas. Next-generation sequencing and polymerase chain technologies have allowed the identification of multiple species-specific bacterial and fungal signatures within granulomas.[16–18] However, the significance of identifying these organisms within granulomas remains to be clarified.

LYMPHOCYTIC OR DIABETIC MASTOPATHY

Lymphocytic mastopathy is an uncommon breast condition that presents with single or multiple clinical masses or mammographic densities. It is thought that the process is probably immune-mediated, as the masses are microscopically associated with dense perilobular and perivascular lymphocytic (mainly B-cell) infiltrates, lobular atrophy, and dense stromal fibrosis.[19] The lymphocytic infiltrate is often accompanied by stromal epithelial myofibroblasts, which can lead to a mistaken diagnosis of invasive carcinoma, granular cell tumor, or Rosai-Dorfman disease. This condition is most common in women with insulin-dependent (type 1) diabetes.[20] However, cases with similar pathologic features may occur in the absence of diabetes mellitus, such as in women with autoimmune thyroid disorders. Thus, a general pathologic term, "sclerosing lymphocytic lobulitis" or "lymphocytic mastopathy," may be preferable to "diabetic mastopathy."[21]

Historical Background for Diabetic Mastopathy

Diabetic mastopathy is an uncommon disease process seen in premenopausal women with long-standing type I diabetes mellitus. The condition was first described by Soler and Khardori in 1984, who studied 12 female patients with insulin-dependent diabetes, limited joint mobility (cheiroarthropathy), thyroiditis, and painless fibrous breast masses.[22] The investigators suggested that because of a relationship between cheiroarthropathy and the effect of hyperglycemia on connective tissue, fibrous breast masses may represent another manifestation of connective tissue disease. They also noted similar appearances between the lymphocytic infiltrates in the fibrous breast masses and those seen in the patients with Hashimoto thyroiditis. In this study, there was no relationship between any human leukocyte antigen histocompatibility subtype and cheiroarthropathy.

In 1987, Byrd and colleagues[23] described the distinct pathologic features of biopsies done for "mastopathy in insulin-dependent diabetics" as dense fibrosis with increased fibroblasts and perivascular lymphocytic infiltrates. Notably, no patients had duct hyperplasia, changes in their epithelial cells, or findings that suggest malignancy. In 1992, Tomaszewski and colleagues[24] coined the term "diabetic mastopathy" and further characterized the pathologic findings of breast masses in patients with long-standing diabetes. They demonstrated that the lymphocytic perivascular infiltrates were composed primarily of B cells and that there was a dense keloid-like fibrosis containing "epithelioid fibroblasts," which appeared to be unique to patients with diabetes. The epithelioid fibroblasts were thought to be an unusual form of myofibroblast known to contain muscle-specific actin and to stain positive for a pan B-cell marker (MB2) on immunostaining studies.

In 2000, Camuto and colleagues[25] proposed 4 diagnostic criteria for diabetic mastopathy: (1) premenopausal woman with long-standing type I diabetes mellitus with associated microvascular complications, such as diabetic retinopathy, neuropathy, or nephropathy; (2) a firm, nontender breast mass identified on clinical breast examination, clinically suspicious for carcinoma; (3) mammographic and ultrasonographic findings of increased density, but without a discrete mass; and (4) excisional or core needle biopsy showing dense keloidal fibrosis associated with periductal or perilobular lymphocytic infiltrate, with or without epithelioid fibroblasts.

Clinical Presentation

Patients with diabetic mastopathy are premenopausal women in their 30s to 40s with insulin-dependent diabetes, who present with one or more painless, well-defined breast masses, although there can be variable examination findings.[25] Although most patients have type I diabetes, there have also been cases reported in patients with type II diabetes. Patients commonly have another complication of long-standing disease, such as nephropathy, neuropathy, or retinopathy. Patients can present with unilateral or bilateral masses and typically do not have lymphadenopathy. Although the masses are benign, they are often clinically indistinguishable from breast cancer on examination or imaging, which leads to core needle or excisional breast biopsies to make a tissue diagnosis. Following initial evaluation, patients can develop recurrences that may be larger in size. In one patient case series, 3 of the 5 patients developed a recurrence, commonly within 1 year of diagnosis.[24]

Several studies have proposed diagnostic criteria for diabetic mastopathy.[24–26] Most of these criteria include a history of long-standing insulin-dependent diabetes mellitus, at least one firm breast mass, imaging showing at least one area of increased density, and a biopsy demonstrating keloidal fibrosis.

Pathophysiology

The pathophysiology of diabetic mastopathy remains incompletely understood and is likely multifactorial. It has been proposed that exogenous insulin use may contribute to the formation of the breast masses, as the affected population is almost universally insulin dependent. Others have proposed that hyperglycemia leads to the production of nonenzymatically glycosylated proteins that resist degradation and accumulate in breast tissues.[25,27,28] These proteins may function as neoantigens, which leads to an autoimmune response, B-cell proliferation similar to that seen in other autoimmune conditions, and eventual cytokine release by macrophages.[24]

Imaging

Because of clinical suspicion for underlying malignancy, patients with diabetic mastopathy frequently require imaging to further elucidate the diagnosis. Mammography and ultrasound are the preferred imaging modalities for excluding malignancy.[29] Mammography demonstrates dense parenchyma without a discrete mass, architectural distortion, or calcifications. Ultrasound reveals ill-defined hypoechoic areas with characteristic acoustic shadowing that is more pronounced than that seen with malignancy, likely secondary to fibrosis.[26] Ultrasound can also be useful for image-guided biopsies and monitoring. Computerized tomography (CT) or MRI are unlikely to add valuable information or change management.[27] Imaging findings are not specific enough to yield a diagnosis; therefore, most patients subsequently undergo biopsy.

Pathologic Features

Because of the fibrotic nature of the masses, fine-needle aspiration often does not provide sufficient tissue for diagnosis.[23,26] Therefore, patients should undergo core needle biopsy and if necessary, subsequent excisional biopsy to make a definitive diagnosis.

Grossly, masses associated with diabetic mastopathy are distinct from the surrounding breast tissue, homogeneous, and firm with a tan-white hue. Microscopic examination reveals dense fibrosis with associated perivascular, periductal, and perilobular lymphocytic infiltrates. Importantly, there is no evidence of hyperplasia or malignancy. As mentioned earlier, Tomaszewski and colleagues[24] described the pathologic findings characteristic of diabetic mastopathy: (1) lymphocytic lobulitis and ductitis with glandular atrophy; (2) lymphocytic/mononuclear perivascular inflammation, predominantly B cell; (3) dense, keloid-like fibrosis; and (4) epithelioid-like fibroblasts. This study was the first to describe epithelioid fibroblasts as rounded epithelioid cells with abundant cytoplasm and oval vesicular nuclei, and the investigators proposed that their presence was pathognomonic of diabetic mastopathy. However, Seidman and colleagues[28] later demonstrated that epithelioid fibroblasts were not essential for the diagnosis of diabetic mastopathy.

Management

Because diabetic mastopathy is a benign condition, not associated with increased risk of subsequent breast cancer, there are no specific interventions recommended after the diagnosis has been confirmed. In most cases, the diagnosis can be made by coupling a high index of suspicion with core needle biopsy, thereby avoiding the need for excisional biopsy. However, the dense fibrosis can make it difficult to obtain enough tissue for accurate diagnosis by core needle biopsy.

At this time, there are no differences in breast cancer screening guidelines for those with diabetic mastopathy compared with women at average risk of developing breast cancer. Patients should be advised that they may develop subsequent breast masses in either breast, even after surgical excision. Because new breast masses could represent breast malignancy, they should not be presumed to be diabetic mastopathy but should undergo standard evaluation with mammogram, ultrasound, and core biopsy, if necessary.

SUMMARY

The operative management of periareolar mastitis consists of central duct excision, excision of the site of the abscess at the periareolar margin, and reconstruction of the subareolar complex.

The investigators' current treatment strategy for granulomatous lobular mastitis avoids surgical procedures in favor of aspiration of abscesses, management with short courses of antibiotics, and even observation for the treatment of milder cases of granulomatous mastitis.

Lymphocytic or diabetic mastopathy occurs in patients with long-standing insulin-dependent diabetes, especially those with microvascular complications such as retinopathy, nephropathy, or neuropathy. Once the diagnosis has been confirmed by core needle biopsy, surgical excision can generally be avoided.

CLINICS CARE POINTS

- When being consulted to manage an erythematous breast, the first consideration is to distinguish routine breast abscess from inflammatory breast cancer, periareolar mastitis, or granulomatous mastitis.
- The pathognomonic findings of periareolar mastitis on clinical examination are the presence of the abscess at the areolar margin and a transverse cleft in the nipple.

- After initial management of periareolar mastitis with fine-needle aspiration and oral antibiotics, a decision must be made on whether central duct excision is necessary.
- Because granulomatous lobular mastitis and diabetic mastopathy have clinical and radiographic features similar to carcinoma of the breast, ultrasound-guided core needle biopsy is essential to establish an accurate diagnosis.

DISCLOSURE

This research did not receive funding from agencies in the public, commercial, or nonprofit sectors.

REFERENCES

1. Urban J. Excision of the major duct system of the breast. Cancer 1963;16: 516–20.
2. Scanlon EF. Breast disease, benign diseases of the breast. In: McKenna RJ, Murphy GP, editors. Fundamentals of surgical oncology. New York: Macmillan Publishing Company; 1986. p. 553–4.
3. Lannin DR. Twenty-two year experience with recurring subareolar abscess and lactiferous duct fistula treated by a single breast surgeon. Am J Surg 2004; 188:407–10.
4. Habif DV, Perzin KH, Lipton R, et al. Subareolar abscess associated with squamous metaplasia of lactiferous ducts. Am J Surg 1970;119:523–6.
5. Schafer P, Furrer C, Mermillod B. An association of cigarette smoking with recurrent subareolar breast abscess. Int J Epidemiol 1988;17:810–3.
6. Olimpiadi YB, Brownson KE, Ding L, et al. Outcomes from treatment of granulomatous lobular mastitis. Surg Pract Sci 2021. https://doi.org/10.1016/j.sipas.2021.100045.
7. Kessler E, Wolloch Y. Granulomatous mastitis: a lesion clinically simulating carcinoma. Am J Clin Pathol 1972;58(6):642–6.
8. Martinez-Ramos D, Simone-Monterde L, Suelves-Piqueres C. Idiopathic granulomatous mastitis: a systematic review of 3060 patients. Breast J 2019;25(6): 1245–50.
9. Davis J Cocco D, Matz S. Re-evaluating if observation continues to be the best management of idiopathic granulomatous mastitis. Surgery 2019;166(6): 1176–80.
10. Korkut E, Akcay MN, Karadeniz E. Granulomatous mastitis: a ten-year experience at a university hospital. Eurasian J Med 2015;47(3):165–73.
11. Brownson KE, Bertoni DM, Lannin DR. Granulomatous lobular mastitis-another paradigm shift in treatment. Breast J 2019;25(4):790–1.
12. Kaviani A, Noveiry BB, Jamei K, et al. How to manage idiopathic granulomatous mastitis: suggestion of an algorithm. Breast J 2014;20(1):110–2.
13. Freeman CM, Xia BT, Wilson GC. Idiopathic granulomatous mastitis: a diagnostic and therapeutic challenge. Am J Surg 2017;214(4):701–6.
14. Jayia P, Oberg E, Tuffaha H. Should we manage all cases of granulomatous mastits conservatively? A 14-year experience. Breast J 2013;19(2):215–6.
15. Aghajanzadeh M, Hassanzadeh R, Alizadeh Sefat S. Granulomatous mastitis: presentations, diagnosis, treatment and outcome in 206 patients from the north of Iran. Breast 2015;24(4):456–60.

16. Ma Naik, Korlimaria A, Shetty ST. Cystic neutrophilic granulomatous mastitis: a clinicopathological study with 16s rRNA sequencing for the detection of corynebacterial in formalin-fixed paraffin embedded tissue. Int J Surg Pathol 2020;28(4): 371–8.
17. Wang J, Xu H, Li Z. Pathogens in patients with granulomatous lobular mastitis. J Infect Dis 2019;81:123–7.
18. Yu HJ, Deng H, Ma J. Clinical metagenomic analysis of bacterial communities in breast abscess of granulomatous mastitis. Int J Infect Dis 2016;53:30–3.
19. Collins LC. Section 7. Breast. In: Goldblum JR, Lamps LW, McKenney JK, et al, editors. Rosai and ackerman's surgical pathology. 11th Edition. Philadelphia: Elsevier, Inc; 2018. p. 1434–527.
20. Lester SC. Chapter 23. The Breast. In: Kumar V, Abbas AK, Aster JC, editors. Robbins and cotran pathologic basis of disease. 9th Edition. Philadelphia: Elsevier, Inc; 2015. p. 1043–72.
21. Ellis IO, Lee AHS, Pinder SE, et al. Volume 2, Chapter 16. Tumors of the breast. In: Fletcher CDM, editor. Diagnostic histopathology of tumors. 5th Edition. Philadelphia: Elsevier, Inc; 2021. p. 1119–210.
22. Soler NG, Khardori R. Fibrous disease of the breast, thyroiditis, and cheiroarthropathy in type I diabetes mellitus. Lancet 1984;1(8370):193–5.
23. Byrd BF Jr, Hartmann WH, Graham LS, et al. Mastopathy in insulin-dependent diabetics. Ann Surg 1987;205(5):529–32.
24. Tomaszewski JE, Brooks JS, Hicks D, et al. Diabetic mastopathy: a distinctive clinicopathologic entity. Hum Pathol 1992;23(7):780–6.
25. Camuto PM, Zetrenne E, Ponn T. Diabetic mastopathy: a report of 5 cases and a review of the literature. Arch Surg 2000;135(10):1190–3.
26. Logan WW, Hoffman NY. Diabetic fibrous breast disease. Radiology 1989;172(3): 667–70.
27. Thorncroft K, Forsyth L, Desmond S, et al. The diagnosis and management of diabetic mastopathy. Breast J 2007;13(6):607–13.
28. Seidman JD, Schnaper LA, Phillips LE. Mastopathy in insulin-requiring diabetes mellitus. Hum Pathol 1994;25(8):819–24.
29. Andrews-Tang D, Diamond AB, Rogers L, et al. Diabetic mastopathy: adjunctive use of ultrasound and utility of core biopsy in diagnosis. Breast J 2000;6(3): 183–8.

Management of Stromal Lesions

Jingjing Yu, MD[a], Kari Kansal, MD[b],*

KEYWORDS

- Fibroepithelial lesions • Fibroadenoma • Phyllodes tumor • PASH
- Periductal stromal tumor

KEY POINTS

- The majority of stromal lesions are benign.
- Benign phyllodes tumors, in contrast to borderline or malignant tumors, may be excised and followed.
- PASH may be followed after diagnosis with core biopsy.

INTRODUCTION

The management of breast stromal lesions requires a multidisciplinary approach utilizing surgery, pathology, and breast imaging. Previously, patients with a breast mass underwent excision without a thorough workup to determine optimal treatment. This article discusses breast stromal lesions including fibroadenomas, phyllodes tumors, pseudoangiomatous stromal hyperplasia, periductal stromal tumors, and lipomas with respect to diagnosis and management.

FIBROADENOMAS
Background

Fibroadenomas are the most common benign mass in women under the age of 30 and account for approximately 68% of benign breast lesions.[1] Comprised of both epithelial and stromal components, they arise from the lobules of the breast and can be either intracanalicular or pericanalicular (**Fig. 1**B). While the exact etiology of fibroadenomas is unknown, hormonal stimulation is thought to play a role as they are commonly found during reproductive years, grow during pregnancy, involute after menopause, and may also be found in postmenopausal women on hormone replacement therapy.[2]

[a] 333 City Boulevard West, Suite 700, Orange, CA 92868, USA; [b] Department of Surgery, University of California, Irvine, Orange, CA, USA
* Corresponding author. 333 City Boulevard West, Suite 700, Orange, CA 92868.
E-mail address: kkansal@hs.uci.edu
Twitter: @Dr_KariKansal (K.K.)

Surg Clin N Am 102 (2022) 1017–1030
https://doi.org/10.1016/j.suc.2022.07.002
0039-6109/22/© 2022 Elsevier Inc. All rights reserved.

surgical.theclinics.com

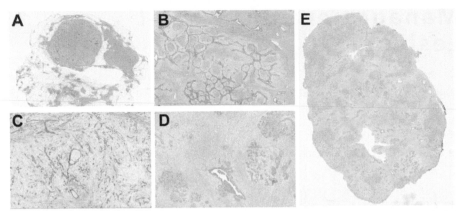

Fig. 1. Histological sections of fibroadenoma lesions. (*A*). Well circumscribed fibroepithelial mass composed of compressed ducts and fibrous stroma. (*B*). High power view of proliferative fibrous stroma compressing breast ducts (intracanalicular pattern). (*C*). Typical fibroadenoma showing loose fibrous stroma and cellularity. (*D*). Fibroadenoma with bland hypercellular stroma component, no stromal atypia is identified. (*E*). Lower power view of hypercellular fibroadenoma.

Presentation/pathology

Fibroadenomas typically present in premenopausal women in their 20s and 30s, although they can be found at any age.[3] Approximately 15 to 20% of patients will have multiple fibroadenomas on presentation[4,5] and 10% are bilateral. The most common type of fibroadenoma is simple fibroadenoma which typically presents as a smooth, mobile, painless, well-defined mass in the breast. Juvenile fibroadenomas are those presenting in women between the age of 10–18 and tend to have more glandularity with greater stromal cellularity. The actual incidence is unknown as many of these masses are not palpable and do not undergo tissue sampling.[6,7] A giant fibroadenoma is greater than 5 cm in size, 500 grams in weight, or displaces at least 4/5 of the breast tissue. These are most often found in adolescent patients.[8] Complex fibroadenomas are associated with cysts, sclerosing adenosis, epithelial calcifications, or papillary apocrine metaplasia.[9] While fibroadenomas do not undergo malignant change, these complex lesions confer a slightly increased risk of future breast cancer when multicentric proliferative changes are noted on biopsy in the surrounding glandular tissue.

Diagnosis

Patients with fibroadenomas present with either a mass on physical exam or are found incidentally on breast imaging. If a patient presents with a new breast mass, triple assessment (physical exam, breast imaging, and core biopsy) should be performed. Mammogram will demonstrate a well-defined round, oval or lobulated mass (**Fig. 2A**).[10] Ultrasound (US) will demonstrate a well-demarcated, smooth, wider than tall, hypoechoic mass (**Fig. 2B**).[11] Breast magnetic resonance imaging (MRI) is rarely used in the setting of a benign breast mass, but if an MRI has been performed and a fibroadenoma is noted, it will classically demonstrate progressive contrast enhancement with nonenhancing internal septations (**Fig. 2C**).

Diagnosis of a fibroadenoma is clear at the time of core biopsy or excision (**Fig. 1**). If the diagnosis is not clear at core biopsy and shows a cellular fibroadenoma or

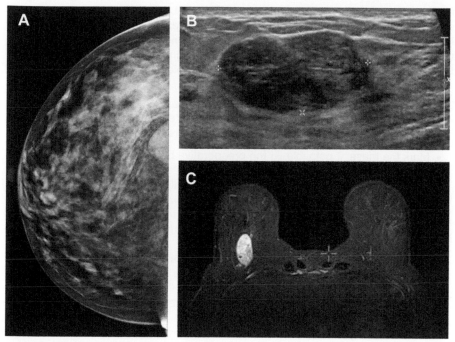

Fig. 2. Radiographic images of fibroadenoma. (*A*). Craniocaudal mammogram of the right breast demonstrates a partially imaged, circumscribed mass at posterior depth. (*B*). Focused ultrasound demonstrates an oval, circumscribed, hypoechoic mass, nonspecific in appearance but typical of a fibroadenoma. (*C*). Axial contrast-enhanced MRI demonstrates an oval, circumscribed enhancing mass with low-signal, nonenhancing internal septations, also characteristic of a fibroadenoma.

fibroepithelial lesion (**Fig. 1**D–E), complete excision is recommended as these can also be seen with a phyllodes tumor.

Management

The management of fibroadenoma falls into 2 categories: observation and surgical excision. In addition to these 2 categories, some fibroadenomas can be treated with minimally invasive techniques including cryoablation, radiofrequency ablation and US-guided percutaneous excision. Due to the benign natural history of simple fibroadenomas, those under 2 cm can be observed once the diagnosis is made using a core needle biopsy. These patients should return for a breast US in 3–6 months to evaluate the mass for growth. If it remains stable, no further follow-up is required and the patient may represent for evaluation if any change in the size of the mass is noted. Small fibroadenomas are generally excised if core biopsy reveals a complex fibroadenoma or fibroepithelial lesion (**Fig. 1**D–E). These are removed regardless of size to rule out phyllodes tumor.

If the fibroadenoma is over 2 cm at presentation, or is noted on follow-up imaging to be enlarging, excision is recommended. Excision is recommended for large and enlarging fibroadenomas as they can become unappealing from a cosmetic standpoint, symptomatic (pain), and/or require a large incision to remove the mass. There is no risk of malignant transformation if it is not resected. Importantly, excision is recommended for all giant fibroadenomas to rule out a phyllodes tumor. Juvenile fibroadenomas should also be excised at the time of diagnosis as they are prone to rapid growth. Care should be taken to preserve breast tissue in an adolescent as this can cause damage to developing breast parenchyma as well as the nipple–areolar complex. The use of surgical excision to diagnose and treat a juvenile fibroadenoma may be preferable to avoid the trauma of a biopsy in this patient population.[8]

Excision

Most benign masses in the breast can be followed or excised in an outpatient setting. The key steps to excision of a benign breast mass are as follows:

- Mark the mass, if palpable, in the preoperative holding area with the patient to ensure the correct mass is being removed.
- If the mass is not palpable, use preoperative localization to ensure accurate identification of the mass.
- Incision placement should be chosen based on the surgeon's comfort and location of the target area. Many times, the areola or inframammary fold can be used to hide the scar.
- After infiltration of local anesthetic, the surgeon should dissect directly the mass being excised. In the benign setting, there is no need to remove healthy breast tissue.
- The incision should be closed in layers and local anesthetic infused for patient comfort.
- This is typically an outpatient procedure.

Minimally invasive techniques

The move toward less invasive techniques in benign breast masses gives patients the opportunity to treat their mass with minimal recovery time without a scar. Cryoablation has been used to treat biopsy-proven fibroadenomas. A group from the University of Washington treated fibroadenomas 7 to 42 mm in size in an ambulatory setting utilizing a two-freeze cycle. The tumors showed shrinkage over 3–12 months.[12] US-guided percutaneous excision has been used in benign breast lesions up to 3 cm in diameter. Grady and colleagues followed 52 patients after percutaneous excision where all visible pieces were removed. The overall recurrence rate was 15% and all recurrences were in lesions larger than 2 cm in size at presentation. They conclude that if the lesion is less than 2 cm at presentation, they do not need further treatment or surveillance.[13] Overall complication rate of US-guided percutaneous excision is slightly higher than surgical excision and there is a risk of incomplete removal, but the advantages are minimal residual scar, excellent cosmesis and a safe alternative to the operating room for benign masses.[5] Lastly, percutaneous radiofrequency-assisted excision of fibroadenomas has also been utilized. Compared to cryoablation and percutaneous biopsy radiofrequency assisted excision allows for adequate sampling for histopathology and margin analysis.[14,15] These modalities are not currently favored among the majority of breast surgeons but there may be an increasing role for these techniques in the future.

SUMMARY

Fibroadenomas are the most commonly diagnosed benign mass in women, often occurring in younger women. Many can be observed once the diagnosis has been made, but if growing or over 2 cm may be treated safely with surgical excision or a percutaneous approach.

CLINICAL CARE POINTS

- All new breast masses must be evaluated with breast exam, imaging, and histopathology.
- Fibroadenomas are a benign breast mass and are not a high-risk lesion for breast cancer, although complex fibroadenomas portend a slightly increased risk of a future breast cancer.
- If excised, all approaches can be conducted as an outpatient with minimal downtime.

PHYLLODES TUMORS
Background

Phyllodes tumors are a rare, biphasic, fibroepithelial tumor of the breast making up 0.3–0.5% of all breast neoplasms.[16] Phyllodes tumors were initially labeled "cystosar-coma phyllodes" by Johanes Muller in 1838, who used the term "sarcoma" based on the fleshy appearance of the tumor.[17] The first case of metastatic phyllodes tumor was identified in 1931.[18] The neutral term "phyllodes tumor" was coined by World Health Organization in 1981 to denote the diverse behavior of these tumors.[19] They are sub-categorized as benign, borderline and malignant based on multiple histologic features and have a diverse behavior from benign and locally recurrent to malignant and met-astatic. The overall prognosis and recurrence rate vary by the category of the phyl-lodes tumor. The average annual incidence rate for malignant phyllodes tumors is 2.1 per million women and is noted to be higher in Latina women compared to other ethnicities.[20]

Presentation

Phyllodes tumors commonly present as a quickly growing palpable solitary mass in the breast and at the time of diagnosis are often greater than 3 cm in size. They are often painless, but can grow large enough to cause attenuation or ulceration of the skin. The presenting symptoms of differing types of phyllodes tumor are similar, and both benign and malignant phyllodes tumors can present at a late stage. While they can occur at any age, they are most common in women in their fifth decade of life.[21] It is well established that women with Li-Fraumeni syndrome are at an increased risk of phyllodes tumor and newer data show approximately 10% of women diag-nosed with malignant phyllodes tumors who underwent germline testing had a delete-rious mutation (BRCA1, BRCA2, RB1, and TP53). At this time, phyllodes tumor diagnosis does not meet National Comprehensive Cancer Network criteria for genetic testing, but this area is undergoing further research.[22]

Diagnosis

Phyllodes tumors usually are seen as focal masses on mammogram, potentially with lobulated margins (**Fig. 3**A).[23] US will demonstrate a well-demarcated, smooth, wider than tall, hypoechoic mass with a vascular flow (**Fig. 3**B). Breast MRI may be used to demonstrate the extent of disease and invasion into surrounding struc-tures. Variations in all of the above imaging may occur, therefore, tissue diagnosis is important.

Core needle biopsy will include the histologic structure needed to characterize the phyllodes tumor as benign, borderline or malignant (**Fig. 4**). It should be noted that fine needle aspiration has been shown to be nondiagnostic in the diagnosis of phyllodes tumor.[24] Diagnosis of phyllodes tumor with the histologic characterization will drive treatment, prognosis, and risk of recurrence. Characterization is based on stromal

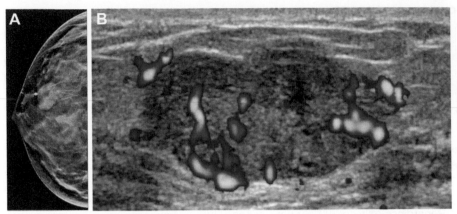

Fig. 3. Radiographic images of phyllodes tumor. (*A*). Craniocaudal mammogram of the right breast shows an oval with lobulated margins at anterior depth. (*B*). Focused ultrasound shows an oval, hypoechoic mass that is wider than tall with internal blood flow on power Doppler interrogation.

atypia, stromal cellularity, stromal overgrowth, mitotic count, and tumor border (**Table 1**). Classification of these tumors is challenging as the assessment of each histologic parameter has not been standardized and it remains unclear which histological features are most predictive of behavior.[25]

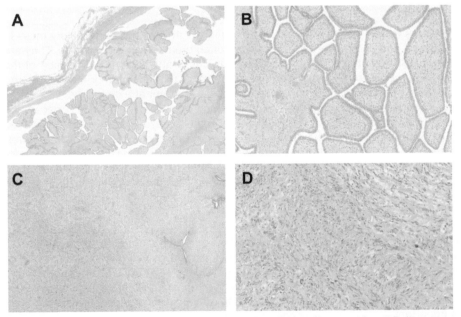

Fig. 4. Histological sections of phyllodes lesions. (*A*). Benign lesion with epithelium overlying cellular fibrous stroma; displays broad leaf-like architecture. (*B*). High power view of benign lesion with leaf-like architecture and bland stroma cells. (*C*). Malignant hypercellular spindle cell lesion with atypia and mitosis and multiple foci of stromal overgrowth. (*D*). High power view of malignant lesion with markedly atypical stromal cells, stromal hypercellularity, and abundant mitotic figures.

Table 1
Characterization of phyllodes tumors

	Benign	Borderline	Malignant
Stromal atypia	Mild	Moderate	Marked
Stromal cellularity	Mildly increased	Moderately increased	Markedly and diffusely increased
Stromal overgrowth	Absent	Absent or very focal	Present
Mitotic count	<5/10 HPF or <2.5/mm^2	5–9/10 HPF or 1.5-<5/mm^2	$\geq$ 10/10 HPF or $\geq$ 5/mm^2
Tumor border	Well-defined	Well-defined or focally permeative	Diffusely permeative

Regardless of histologic characterization, a phyllodes tumor has a higher potential for rapid growth and local recurrence than a fibroadenoma which underscores the need for an accurate and timely diagnosis. If a core biopsy cannot be completed at the time of diagnosis, or is not definitive, an excisional biopsy should be performed. Based on the final pathology from excisional biopsy, a patient may need to return to the operating room to obtain a clear margin. Due to this, the preference is to have a histopathological diagnosis prior to surgery although in some cases it is challenging to diagnose a phyllodes tumor on core biopsy.

Management

The management of phyllodes tumors depends on their histologic classification. Surgical excision is recommended for the initial treatment of phyllodes tumors with either breast-conserving surgery or mastectomy. NCCN guidelines recommend all phyllodes tumors be excised with a margin of $\geq$ 1 cm clear margin to decrease the risk of recurrence (NCCN guidelines). Significant research has focused on whether these margins are excessive or inadequate.[26–32] Benign phyllodes tumors treated with enucleation without a negative margin have an acceptable recurrence rate.[22] A wider negative margin did not reduce the risk of recurrence which supports the treatment of benign phyllodes tumors with an excisional biopsy rather than a wide local excision (negative margin greater than 1 cm). However, it should be noted this is not congruent with current NCCN guidelines. For borderline or malignant phyllodes tumors, excision with greater than 1 cm margin remains the standard of care. In most cases, the masses are very large at diagnosis and require mastectomy to obtain adequate margins.

Phyllodes tumors spread primarily via a hematogenous route, and rarely involve regional lymph nodes so routine lymph node evaluation is not recommended.[33–35] In the setting of a borderline or malignancy phyllodes tumor, staging with a chest x-ray or chest CT and consideration of an abdominal CT are recommended to rule out metastatic spread to the lungs and liver.

Postoperative radiotherapy does not routinely play a role in the treatment of malignant phyllodes tumors and there is no role in benign phyllodes tumors. Radiation has been used to decrease regional recurrence in the setting of a chest wall recurrence, or with inadequate margins in borderline and malignant phyllodes tumors but has no effect on overall survival or distant-free survival.[36,37] Radiation therapy remains controversial as studies have yet shown consistent beneficial outcomes. These cases should be discussed in a multidisciplinary tumor board to evaluate the benefit of adjuvant radiation in individual patients.

Systemic therapy has a limited role and is used as palliation in the metastatic setting. Preferred chemotherapeutic agents include: ifosfamide, cisplatin, etoposide, or doxorubicin.[38] Newer agents are looking at the role of molecular targeting agents including tyrosine kinase inhibitors. Due to the poor prognosis and survival once a patient is metastatic, they should pursue clinical trial inclusion and investigational medications.

Outcomes

Long terms outcomes for benign phyllodes tumors are excellent. There is a low risk of a local recurrence after excision.[28–32] Women younger than 25 are at an increased risk of recurrence compared to older patients.[39] These patients should be followed with breast US every 6 months for 3 years. If a recurrence is noted, re-excision is recommended. In those that recur there is a 20% histologic upgrade.[25]

Borderline and malignant phyllodes tumors have a local recurrence rate ranging from 10 to 65%.[40] Spanheimer and colleagues evaluated a single institution's experience with borderline and malignant phyllodes tumors to evaluate factors associated with increased risk of recurrence. They found those who were younger than 40 and had close/positive margins were at an associated increased risk. Those patients with uniformly poor pathologic features including marked stromal atypia, stromal overgrowth, infiltrative borders, and 10 or more mitoses per 10 high-powered fields (HPF) were most likely to have a distant recurrence and poor overall prognosis. Those without uniformly poor histologic features had a 10-year disease-specific survival of 100%.[40] Approximately 25% of malignancy phyllodes tumors metastasize to the lungs, bone, liver, and brain. The overall survival is poor with the majority of patients dying within three years of diagnosis.[39,41]

SUMMARY

Phyllodes tumors are rare and present with a quickly enlarging breast mass. They have a wide range of outcomes based on histologic characterization. The mainstay of treatment remains surgical excision at the time of diagnosis and data suggest benign phyllodes tumors can be enucleated rather than removed with a wide negative margin.

CLINICAL CARE POINTS

- All phyllodes tumors must be treated with excision. Borderline and malignant tumors require a wide negative margin greater than 1 cm to decrease the risk of recurrence.
- Adjuvant radiation and systemic therapy for malignant phyllodes tumors show variable outcomes and require further investigation.
- Metastatic phyllodes tumors have a poor outcome and effort should be made for patients to be placed on clinical trial and treated in a multidisciplinary setting.

PSEUDOANGIOMATOUS STROMAL HYPERPLASIA
Background and histology

Pseudoangiomatous stromal hyperplasia (PASH), first described by Vuitch and colleagues[42] in 1986 is a benign breast lesion of mesenchymal origin. It is characterized histologically by the proliferation of breast stroma with inter-anastomosing slit--like channels lined by myofibroblasts. These resemble vascular structures but are not lined by endothelial cells and do not contain red blood cells, hence the term "pseudoangiomatous" (**Fig. 5**A).[44] PASH is positive for estrogen, progesterone and androgen receptors, CD34, and vimentin. It is negative for CD31 and factor VIII, which are endothelial markers that distinguish PASH from angiosarcoma.[45]

Presentation

There is a wide spectrum of clinical presentations for PASH. In a study by Jones and colleagues[46] of 57 patients, 53% patients presented with an abnormality seen on screening mammography, 44% presented with palpable abnormalities, and 3% had PASH incidentally detected on evaluation for different abnormalities. Additionally, cases of bilateral breast involvement with rapid enlargement of the breasts have also been reported.[43,47,48] PASH is typically diagnosed in perimenopausal women but has also been reported in men with gynecomastia and in menopausal women on hormone replacement therapy.[47,49] Given these patterns of presentation, PASH is thought to result from hormonal stimuli.[45,49]

Diagnosis

There are no distinct imaging features pathognomonic for PASH, and differentiation of PASH from other stromal lesions such as fibroadenoma can be challenging. On mammography, PASH often presents as a well-circumscribed mass, although irregular margins may be appreciated. US may demonstrate circumscribed, hypoechoic or heterogeneous masses with or without posterior shadowing (**Fig. 5**B). MRI may reveal numerous masses with reticular and cystic change in T2 weighted sequences, with rapid and persistent or progressive enhancement. In cases with diffuse bilateral breast involvement, PASH can be seen as diffuse bilateral enhancement or as large masses with persistent enhancement on postcontrast sequences.[10,23,44,50] Core needle biopsy is required to confirm the diagnosis.

Management

The management of PASH varies from observation to surgical intervention. If imaging and pathology findings are consistent with PASH, the lesion can be observed as PASH itself is a benign entity. Excision can be considered if there are suspicious findings on imaging to suggest the coexistence of PASH with malignant lesions. Excision may also be considered if the patient has a strong family history of breast cancer, is symptomatic, or has an enlarging lesion.[45]

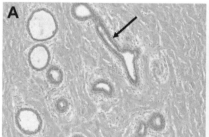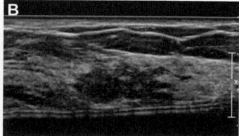

Fig. 5. Pseudoangiomatous stromal tumor. (*A*). Histological section shows breast stroma composed of dense collagenase tissue with complex anastomosing spaces (*arrow*) lined with myofibroblasts. (*B*). Ultrasound demonstrates an irregular, hypoechoic mass with spiculated margins and a hyperechoic halo of surrounding tissue.

PERIDUCTAL STROMAL TUMORS
Background and histology

Periductal stromal tumors (PST) are a rare, low-grade neoplasm accounting for less than 1% of breast malignancies.[51] They are biphasic lesions, meaning they have benign ducts surrounded by sarcomatous stroma. They also lack leaf-like architecture, making them distinguishable and characterized separately from phyllode tumors.[52–54] The histologic criteria for PST as determined by the Armed Forces Institute of Pathology are as follows:[55]

1. Predominately sarcomatous stromal proliferation around benign ducts devoid of leaf-like growth pattern
2. One or more nodules separated by adipose tissue
3. Stomal mitotic activity $\geq$3/10 high power fields
4. Stromal infiltration into surrounding adipose tissue

By immunohistochemistry, PST is positive for CD34 and CD10 but negative for estrogen and progesterone receptors.[53]

Presentation

PST is more common in perimenopausal and postmenopausal women. In a study by Burga and colleagues of 20 PST cases from the Armed Forces Institute of Pathology Histology, the median age was 55.3 years old, 10 years older than those presenting with phyllodes tumor. PST can present as a single nodule or multinodular tumor with reported mass size ranging from 0.2 to 20 cm.[51,55]

Diagnosis

There is a paucity of known radiographic features for PST given its rare occurrence. In one report by Ding and colleagues, the authors described the radiologic features of a PST by multiple modalities. US revealed multiple hypoechoic and heterogenous masses with internal septations and abundant blood flow on color Doppler imaging. Mammography and digital breast tomosynthesis showed multiple lobulated high-density masses comprising almost the entire right breast.[51] However, it is important to note the imaging findings of phyllodes and PST overlap, and histopathologic evaluation is required for definitive diagnosis.

Management

The management of PST requires surgical resection. Given the infiltrative nature of PST and risk of recurrence, achieving negative margins is recommended. Adjuvant chemotherapy and radiation are not recommended.[53]

There is also evidence PST can transform into sarcoma. Burga and colleagues reported one patient from their study had PST with a component of high-grade angiosarcoma on pathology. Another patient had a recurrence 5 years later with pathology revealing phyllodes architecture, suggesting the progression of PST to phyllodes tumor over time.[55] Additional surgical resection including mastectomy may be required for recurrence.[55]

BREAST LIPOMA

Lipoma of the breast is a benign tumor comprised of mature fat cells. Clinically, it presents as a well-circumscribed, mobile, painless mass.[56] Lipomas are usually small but there have also been reports of giant lipomas over 10 cm or 1000g.[57,58] The incidence of lipomas is unclear in the literature, with Donegan reporting an incidence of 2.2%

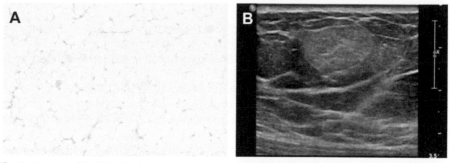

Fig. 6. Lipoma. (*A*). Histological section shows mature adipocytes without atypia. (*B*). Ultrasound demonstrates a round, hyperechoic mass with circumscribed margins, typical in appearance for a lipoma.

while another report found histologically verified lipomas in 4.6% of excision biopsy specimens.[59]

There are challenges to diagnosing lipoma of the breast. Fine needle aspiration may reveal only fat cells, which is considered inadequate by definition, or fat and epithelial cells which may cast doubt on the diagnosis.[59] At mammography, lipomas are seen as well-circumscribed, fat-containing masses. They can have varying echogenicity on US without vascularity on color Doppler interrogation. The characteristic appearance of breast lipoma is a fat-containing mass at mammography corresponding to an echogenic mass with circumscribed margins on US (**Fig. 6**B).[50] However, both mammography and US scanning are often negative, especially if the lesion is small. In a study by Lanng and colleagues,[59] of 108 women with clinically diagnosed lipomas, mammography, and US only revealed lipoma in 3.0% and 21.0% of cases, respectively.

Given the challenges of diagnosing a breast lipoma, Lanng proposed an approach to diagnosis that includes: clinical diagnosis, core needle biopsy, and lack of suspicious findings at mammogram and US if a lipoma is not demonstrated. If these criteria are met, then observation is reasonable. Excision can be considered if there is diagnostic uncertainty or the mass is enlarging or causing cosmetic deformity.[59] Final histology for lipoma will show mature adipocytes without atypia (**Fig. 6**A).

SUMMARY

Breast stromal lesions are diagnosed on physical exam or breast imaging. It is important to obtain a histopathologic diagnosis prior to determining the role of surgery. Minimally invasive techniques are currently being evaluated but have not been widely accepted. Margins are determined by the pathology of the lesion and conservative management with observation is indicated for certain tumors.

ACKNOWLEDGMENTS

We would like to acknowledge multiple colleagues who contributed to this book article. Dr. Ifegwo Ibe for his contribution of pathology images and descriptions. Dr. Freddie Combs for his contribution to radiology images and descriptions. Dr. Karen Todd Lane and Dr. Nikhil Kansal for offering editing insight and expertise.

DISCLOSURE

The authors have nothing to disclose.

REFERENCES

1. Neinstein LS. Breast disease in adolescents and young women. Pediatr Clin North Am 1999;46(3):607–29.
2. Meyer JE, Frenna TH, Polger M, et al. Enlarging occult fibroadenomas. Radiology 1992;183(3):639–41.
3. Dent DM, Cant PJ. Fibroadenoma. World J Surg 1989;13(6):706–10.
4. Grouthier V, Chakhtoura Z, Tejedor I, et al. Positive association between progestins and the evolution of multiple fibroadenomas in 72 women. Endocr Connect 2020;9(6):570–7.
5. Wang WJ, Wang Q, Cai QP, et al. Ultrasonographically guided vacuum-assisted excision for multiple breast masses: non-randomized comparison with conventional open excision. J Surg Oncol 2009;100(8):675–80.
6. Sanchez R, Ladino-Torres MF, Bernat JA, et al. Breast fibroadenomas in the pediatric population: common and uncommon sonographic findings. Pediatr Radiol 2010;40(10):1681–9.
7. Sanders LM, Sharma P, El Madany M, et al. Clinical breast concerns in low-risk pediatric patients: practice review with proposed recommendations. Pediatr Radiol 2018;48(2):186–95.
8. Sosin M, Pulcrano M, Feldman ED, et al. Giant juvenile fibroadenoma: a systematic review with diagnostic and treatment recommendations. Gland Surg 2015; 4(4):312–21.
9. Nassar A, Visscher DW, Degnim AC, et al. Complex fibroadenoma and breast cancer risk: a Mayo Clinic Benign Breast Disease Cohort Study. Breast Cancer Res Treat 2015;153(2):397–405.
10. Goel NB, Knight TE, Pandey S, et al. Fibrous lesions of the breast: imaging-pathologic correlation. Radiographics 2005;25(6):1547–59.
11. Fornage BD, Lorigan JG, Andry E. Fibroadenoma of the breast: sonographic appearance. Radiology 1989;172(3):671–5.
12. Kaufman CS, Bachman B, Littrup PJ, et al. Office-based ultrasound-guided cryoablation of breast fibroadenomas. Am J Surg 2002;184(5):394–400.
13. Grady I, Gorsuch H, Wilburn-Bailey S. Long-term outcome of benign fibroadenomas treated by ultrasound-guided percutaneous excision. Breast J 2008;14(3):275–8.
14. Fine RE, Staren ED. Percutaneous radiofrequency-assisted excision of fibroadenomas. Am J Surg 2006;192(4):545–7.
15. Li P, Zhang Z, Qin S, et al. The diagnosis of mesenteric fibromatosis: a 90-month five patients case report. J Cancer Res Ther 2016;12(4):1318–20.
16. Rowell MD, Perry RR, Hsiu JG, et al. Phyllodes tumors. Am J Surg 1993;165(3):376–9.
17. Calhoun K, Allison K, Kim J. Chapter 62: phyllodes tumors. Diseases of the breast. 5th Edition. Philadelphia, PA: Lippincott-Williams & Wilkins; 2014.
18. Lee BJ, Pack GT. Giant intracanalicular fibro-adenomyxoma of the breast. The so-called cystosarcoma phyllodes mammae of Johannes Müller. Am J Cancer 1931; 15(4):2583–609.
19. World Health Organization (1981). Histological typing of breast tumours, 2nd ed. World Health Organization.
20. Bernstein L, Deapen D, Ross RK. The descriptive epidemiology of malignant cystosarcoma phyllodes tumors of the breast. Cancer 1993;71(10):3020–4. https://doi.org/10.1002/1097-0142(19930515)71:10<3020::aid-cncr2820711022>3.0.co;2-g.

21. Oberman HA. Cystosarcoma phyllodes; a clinicopathologic study of hypercellular periductal stromal neoplasms of breast. Cancer 1965;18:697–710.
22. Rosenberger LH, Thomas SM, Nimbkar SN, et al. Germline genetic mutations in a multi-center contemporary cohort of 550 phyllodes tumors: an opportunity for expanded multi-gene panel testing. Ann Surg Oncol 2020;27(10):3633–40.
23. Irshad A, Ackerman SJ, Pope TL, et al. Rare breast lesions: correlation of imaging and histologic features with WHO classification. Radiographics 2008;28(5): 1399–414.
24. Krishnamurthy S, Ashfaq R, Shin HJ, et al. Distinction of phyllodes tumor from fibroadenoma: a reappraisal of an old problem. Cancer 2000;90(6):342–9.
25. Tan PH, Thike AA, Tan WJ, et al. Predicting clinical behaviour of breast phyllodes tumours: a nomogram based on histological criteria and surgical margins. J Clin Pathol 2012;65(1):69–76.
26. Barrio AV, Clark BD, Goldberg JI, et al. Clinicopathologic features and long-term outcomes of 293 phyllodes tumors of the breast. Ann Surg Oncol 2007;14(10): 2961–70.
27. Yom CK, Han W, Kim SW, et al. Reappraisal of conventional risk stratification for local recurrence based on clinical outcomes in 285 resected phyllodes tumors of the breast. Ann Surg Oncol 2015;22(9):2912–8.
28. Adesoye T, Neuman HB, Wilke LG, et al. Current trends in the management of phyllodes tumors of the breast. Ann Surg Oncol 2016;23(10):3199–205.
29. Moo T-A, Alabdulkareem H, Tam A, et al. Association between recurrence and re-excision for close and positive margins versus observation in patients with benign phyllodes tumors. Ann Surg Oncol 2017;24(10):3088–92.
30. Park H-L, Kwon S-H, Chang SY, et al. Long-term follow-up result of benign phyllodes tumor of the breast diagnosed and excised by ultrasound-guided vacuum-assisted breast biopsy. J Breast Cancer 2012;15(2):224–9.
31. Qian Y, Quan ML, Ogilvi T, et al. Surgical management of benign phyllodes tumours of the breast: Is wide local excision really necessary? Can J Surg 2018; 61(6):430.
32. Barth R J. Margin negative, breast conserving resection: adequate for benign phyllodes tumors, but inadequate therapy for borderline and malignant phyllodes tumors. Breast Cancer Res Treat 2013;142(2):463–4.
33. Cheng SP, Chang YC, Liu TP, et al. Phyllodes tumor of the breast: the challenge persists. World J Surg 2006;30(8):1414–21.
34. Zurrida S, Bartoli C, Galimberti V, et al. Which therapy for unexpected phyllode tumour of the breast? Eur J Cancer 1992;28(2–3):654–7.
35. Guillot E, Couturaud B, Reyal F, et al. Management of phyllodes breast tumors. Breast J 2011;17(2):129–37.
36. Barth RJ Jr, Wells WA, Mitchell SE, et al. A prospective, multi-institutional study of adjuvant radiotherapy after resection of malignant phyllodes tumors. Ann Surg Oncol 2009;16(8):2288–94.
37. Zeng S, Zhang X, Yang D, et al. Effects of adjuvant radiotherapy on borderline and malignant phyllodes tumors: A systematic review and meta-analysis. Mol Clin Oncol 2015;3(3):663–71.
38. Jardim DLF, Conley A, Subbiah V. Comprehensive characterization of malignant phyllodes tumor by whole genomic and proteomic analysis: biological implications for targeted therapy opportunities. Orphanet J Rare Dis 2013;8(1):1–8.
39. Wei J, Tan YT, Cai YC, et al. Predictive factors for the local recurrence and distant metastasis of phyllodes tumors of the breast: a retrospective analysis of 192 cases at a single center. Chin J Cancer 2014;33(10):492–500.

40. Spanheimer PM, Barrio AV. ASO author reflections: malignant/borderline phyllodes tumors without uniformly poor histologic features have an excellent prognosis. Ann Surg Oncol 2019;26(Suppl 3):619–20.

41. Ganesh V, Lee J, Wan BA, et al. Palliative treatment of metastatic phyllodes tumors: a case series. AME Case Rep 2017;1:9.

42. Vuitch MF, Rosen PP, Erlandson RA. Pseudoangiomatous hyperplasia of mammary stroma. Hum Pathol 1986;17(2):185–91.

43. Xu X, Persing SM, Allam O, et al. Management of recurrent bilateral multifocal pseudoangiomatous stromal hyperplasia (PASH). Breast J 2020;26(9):1814–7.

44. Jung HK, Kim W. Bilateral axillary pseudoangiomatous stromal hyperplasia in a premenopausal woman: a case report with imaging findings. J Clin Ultrasound 2022;50(1):43–8.

45. Raj SD, Sahani VG, Adrada BE, et al. Pseudoangiomatous stromal hyperplasia of the breast: multimodality review with pathologic correlation. Curr Probl Diagn Radiol 2017;46(2):130–5.

46. Jones KN, Glazebrook KN, Reynolds C. Pseudoangiomatous stromal hyperplasia: imaging findings with pathologic and clinical correlation. AJR Am J Roentgenol 2010;195(4):1036–42.

47. Tsuda B, Kumaki N, Ishida R, et al. Rare finding of bilateral pseudoangiomatous stromal hyperplasia of the breast: a case report. Tokai J Exp Clin Med 2019; 44(4):73–9.

48. Pruthi S, Reynolds C, Johnson RE, et al. Tamoxifen in the management of pseudoangiomatous stromal hyperplasia. Breast J 2001;7(6):434–9.

49. Yoon KH, Koo B, Lee KB, et al. Optimal treatment of pseudoangiomatous stromal hyperplasia of the breast. Asian J Surg 2020;43(7):735–41.

50. Whorms DS, Fishman MDC, Slanetz PJ. Mesenchymal lesions of the breast: what radiologists need to know. AJR Am J Roentgenol 2018;211(1):224–33.

51. Ding N, Jiang Y, Liu H, et al. Imaging features of breast periductal stromal tumor: a case report. Front Oncol 2021;11:577227.

52. Wabik A, Van Bockstal MR, Berlière M, et al. Periductal stromal tumors and phyllodes tumors represent a spectrum of fibroepithelial lesions: what is in a name? Int J Surg Pathol 2021;29(1):97–101.

53. Askan G, Arıbal E, Ak G, et al. Periductal stromal tumor of the breast: a case report and review of the literature. J Breast Health 2016;12(3):133–6.

54. Fard EV, Zhang S. Periductal stromal tumor of the breast: case report and literature review. Ann Clin Lab Sci 2018;48(6):770–5.

55. Burga AM, Tavassoli FA. Periductal stromal tumor: a rare lesion with low-grade sarcomatous behavior. Am J Surg Pathol 2003;27(3):343–8.

56. Guray M, Sahin AA. Benign breast diseases: classification, diagnosis, and management. Oncologist 2006;11(5):435–49.

57. Li YF, Lv MH, Chen LF, et al. Giant lipoma of the breast: a case report and review of the literature. Clin Breast Cancer 2011;11(6):420–2.

58. Rodriguez LF, Shuster BA, Milliken RG. Giant lipoma of the breast. Br J Plast Surg 1997;50(4):263–5.

59. Lanng C, Eriksen B, Hoffmann J. Lipoma of the breast: a diagnostic dilemma. Breast 2004;13(5):408–11.

Management of Radiographic Lesions of the Breast

Lisa Wiechmann, MD, FACS[a],*, Lauren Canter Friedlander, MD[b]

KEYWORDS

- Mammogram • DBT • Tomosynthesis • Ultrasound • Sonogram • MRI • BI-RADS
- Mass • Enhancement • Calcifications • Asymmetry • Cyst

KEY POINTS

- Imaging modalities
- BI-RADS classification
- Role of percutaneous biopsy
- Concordance

INTRODUCTION

It is important for surgeons to be familiar with the imaging appearances of a variety of breast lesions; these include benign and malignant tumors, systemic diseases (eg, collagen vascular disease, vasculitis, and so on), and metastatic lesions. Interpretation of imaging studies is important in a variety of clinical settings, including standard evaluation of patients in the office, preoperative evaluation, and intraoperative assessment of both in situ lesions with ultrasonography as well as specimen radiography and postoperative changes seen at subsequent imaging.

Mammography, 2D and 3D (better referred to as digital breast tomosynthesis [DBT]) imaging, ultrasonography, MRI, and nuclear imaging are most commonly used in the diagnosis and management of breast disease with several newer techniques also under investigation.

This article reviews imaging modalities, discusses and illustrates a variety of radiographic lesions of the breast, and discusses radiologic-pathologic correlation when applicable. The article summarizes the role of each modality from the surgeon's perspective as the physician responsible for management of the patient's care.

[a] Division of Breast Surgery, Department of Surgery, Columbia University Irving Medical Center, 161 Fort Washington Ave, 10th Floor, New York, NY 10032, USA; [b] Division of Breast Imaging, Department of Radiology, Columbia University Irving Medical Center, 161 Fort Washington Ave, 10th Floor, New York, NY 10032, USA
* Corresponding author.
E-mail address: Lsw2135@cumc.columbia.edu

Surg Clin N Am 102 (2022) 1031–1041
https://doi.org/10.1016/j.suc.2022.06.005
0039-6109/22/© 2022 Elsevier Inc. All rights reserved.
surgical.theclinics.com

HISTORY/BACKGROUND

Wilhelm Röntgen took the first of the many radiographs to be taken over the next 120 years, in November 1895; it was a photograph (the first roentgenogram) of his wife's hand and wedding ring, and he took it by using a photographic plate on the other side of an electron beam tube. Thanks to his invention, orthopedic trauma, as well as penetrating trauma with radio-opaque metal bullets, pins, and other metal objects could be assessed faster than ever before. The technology was brought to the battlefield by Marie Curie (a recent Nobel Prize winner at the time) when she drove a truck with portable x-ray equipment near the battlefields of France during World War 1.

The need for dedicated breast imaging was first described at the 1924 Radiological Society of North America Annual Meeting in Kansas City, Missouri. Malvern Clopton, MD, stated that "early breast cancer cannot be diagnosed by palpation or inspection." Building on this claim, the work of Stafford Warren, MD, and Ira Lockwood, MD, resulted in the first successful application of direct exposure preoperative breast radiography to help predict malignant from benign disease. Robert Egan's seminal textbook on mammography published in 1960 established the nascent discipline of breast radiology. Egan went as far as describing optimal technical and positioning techniques to enable a more widespread adoption of breast imaging. Subsequent major technologic advances in mammography came with the development of first xeromammography and then screen-film mammography in the 1970s. With this came the adoption of uniform-thickness breast compression, specialized views, and reduced radiation dose. An understanding of the value of screening mammography soon followed. In 1973, the landmark results of the Health Insurance Plan of Greater New York randomized clinical trial demonstrated a statistically significant reduction in breast cancer deaths among women offered screening compared with a control group of women who were not offered screening[1]

The American College of Radiology began its Breast Imaging Reporting and Data System (BI-RADS) initiative in response to requests from referring clinicians to standardize reporting of mammography in 1985.[2,3] Since that time, breast imaging has continued to evolve, with the advent of digital mammography and then tomosynthesis, the application of ultrasound imaging to the breast, and the development of physiologic breast imaging including breast MRI and nuclear imaging. The BI-RADS manual has undergone multiple revisions since its inception, and the standardized lexicon of breast imaging terminology has grown even as the fundamental report standardization has remained the same.

IMAGING MODALITIES
Mammography

Mammography refers to the usage of x-rays to generate images of the breast. Currently used mammography techniques include digital 2D imaging and DBT, sometimes referred to as "3D" imaging. A screening mammography is performed in asymptomatic patients at regular intervals to identify clinically occult breast cancer. A diagnostic mammography is obtained in the presence of symptoms or signs (eg, breast lump, nipple discharge, breast pain) or to further investigate an abnormal finding on a screening mammography.

2D digital mammography collects the radiation on an electronic image detector instead of the previously used analogue film; this technique was adopted widely after conclusion of The Digital Mammographic Imaging Screening Trial.[4] This landmark multi-institution study across 33 sites in the United States and Canada demonstrated that for women younger than 50 years, premenopausal and perimenopausal women, and women with heterogeneously dense or extremely dense breasts digital mammography was more accurate than film screen mammography. Additional advantages included prevention of loss of plain films, lower radiation dose,[5] faster needle localization procedures,[6] and correlation of different imaging modalities on the same digital workstation.

DBT imaging of the breasts involves the acquisition of multiple x-ray projections of the breast across an arc. These projections are then reconstructed by the computer into a series of stacked images such that the interpreting physician can scroll through the layers of breast tissue on the workstation. This technique reduces the challenge posed by overlapping breast tissue. Although DBT is sometimes referred to as 3D imaging, the images are not truly 3-dimensional and this is largely a misnomer. The computer can use the data to generate synthetic 2D images and thus eliminate the need for separately acquired 2D images. Performed this way, the radiation dose from a tomosynthesis examination is about equivalent to that of a standard digital 2D mammography, but provides more information. Compared with 2D digital mammography, DBT has been shown to increase the detection of invasive cancers, particularly invasive lobular cancers; decrease the number of recalls for false-positive findings at screening; and increase the percentage of biopsies with positive results. It has been widely adopted in both the screening and diagnostic settings.[7,8]

Breast Ultrasonography

Ultrasonography is a valuable tool in the evaluation of the breast. Unlike mammography, breast ultrasonography does not expose patients to ionizing radiation. Instead, ultrasound devices emit sound waves, and the echoes returning to the handheld transducer generate real-time images that can be used for both screening and diagnostic evaluation.

The addition of breast ultrasonography to mammography for evaluating masses has been shown to improve the specificity of diagnostic evaluation and reduce the number of biopsies with benign findings.[9] Breast ultrasonography has also been used for whole breast screening in the setting of dense breast tissue. Studies have shown that increased breast density is associated with both decreased cancer detection on mammography and an increased risk of breast cancer. In the American College of Radiology Imaging Network protocol 6666 multicenter trial of whole-breast screening ultrasonography in women at somewhat elevated risk, screening ultrasonography yielded an excess of 4.2 cancers per 1000 beyond mammographic findings.[10] Limitations of breast ultrasonography include operator dependence,[11] time to perform the study, and the high rate of false-positive findings at biopsy.[12] Multiple rounds of screening, interpretation by experienced breast radiologists, and updated BI-RADS guidelines for interpretation have reduced the false-positive rate. The development of automated whole breast ultrasound machines has helped to address issues of operator dependence and time.[13]

In the United States, the Mammography Quality Standards Act that regulates mammography now requires that imaging facilities notify women with dense breast tissue via a lay letter of the masking effects of dense tissue on mammography, provide a qualitative assessment of a woman's breast density, and remind her to bring questions to her provider.[14–16]

Despite its widely recognized utility as a screening tool for breast cancer, breast ultrasonography remains an adjunct to and not a replacement for screening mammography, which is the only tool with a long-proven mortality benefit. Even in the era of DBT, supplemental screening breast ultrasonography remains valuable. For average-risk women with dense breast tissue screened with DBT, recent data have shown that supplemental screening breast ultrasonography can find an additional 0.7 to 9.4 cancers per 1000 women.[17]

Breast MRI

MRI is a technology that uses magnets and radio waves to produce detailed cross-sectional images of the body, again without the use of radiation. Contrast-enhanced breast MRI is the most sensitive imaging modality for depicting breast cancer and has been accepted as the primary supplemental method for screening high-risk patients in addition to mammography.[15,18] Breast MRI is currently used in a variety of clinical settings including:

- Enhanced screening of high-risk women (approved for women with > 20% lifetime risk of breast cancer)
- Evaluating select patients with breast cancer (particularly invasive lobular carcinoma) or other high-risk lesions preoperatively (especially in the setting of discordant physical examination and/or dense breast tissue) to assist in surgical planning.[19]
- Evaluating response to neoadjuvant therapy in patients with cancer[20]
- Evaluating patients with pathologic nipple discharge and negative mammographic/sonographic workup
- Evaluating equivocal findings on mammography/sonography in select cases
- Evaluating the integrity of silicone implants (for which no contrast is required)[21]
- Research trials

Tables 1 and 2 summarize breast imaging diagnostic studies and clinical indications (Table 1) and the pros and cons of each modality (Table 2).

EMERGENT IMAGING MODALITIES: A LOOK TO THE FUTURE

- Contrast-enhanced mammography (CEM):

CEM involves the intravenous injection of iodinated contrast material immediately before dual-energy standard mammographic projections are obtained. The radiologist then reviews both standard 2D mammographic images and images highlighting areas of contrast uptake. Like breast MRI, CEM provides both anatomic and physiologic information about the breast. However, it is less expensive and could therefore be made more widely available than breast MRI. Although it has been shown to approach the accuracy of breast MRI, breast MRI has continued to show somewhat greater sensitivity. CEM can be used to resolve equivocal findings on routine mammography, aid in preoperative staging, screen higher-than-average-risk women for breast cancer, and monitor response to neoadjuvant chemotherapy. CEM provides a good alternative for patients who cannot tolerate breast MRI or for whom breast MRI is contraindicated. CEM-guided biopsy systems are not yet widely available but are in development.[22]

- Nuclear imaging of the breast:

Nuclear imaging of the breast involves the intravenous injection of a radiotracer followed by the positioning of the patient in a detector system to create an image highlighting those areas in the breast that are most vascular or metabolically active. There are 2 radiotracers currently in use: gamma-emitting 99mTc-sestamibi and PET with fludeoxyglucose F 18 (18F-FDG). Dedicated breast gamma-camera imaging can be performed with single-detector systems like breast-specific gamma-imaging (BSGI) or with dual head detectors, often called *molecular breast imaging*. Standard

Table 1
Diagnostic studies and clinical indications

	Diagnostic Mammography	Targeted Ultrasonography	MRI	Image-Guided Core Biopsy
Palpable breast lump or focal breast pain < 30 y old	Selectively	Yes	Selectively	Selectively
Palpable breast lump or focal breast pain >/ = 30 y old	Yes	Yes	Selectively	Selectively
Pathologic nipple discharge	Yes (if age 30+)	Yes	If mammography/ ultrasonography negative	Selectively
Palpable axillary adenopathy	Yes (if age 30+)	Yes	If mammography/ ultrasonography negative	Selectively
Abnormal screening mammogram	If requested by the interpreting radiologist	If requested by the interpreting radiologist	Selectively	Selectively

craniocaudal and mediolateral oblique images are obtained and evaluated alongside standard mammographic images. Positron emission mammography is performed with the injection of 18F-FDG and similar mammographic-style positioning within a detection device. As the technology has improved, studies have shown sensitivity of these nuclear imaging studies similar to that shown by breast MRI with higher specificity. The greatest challenges continue to be dose reduction and reduction in the lengthy study times. At present, direct biopsy is only available with BSGI systems, although biopsy devices for other systems are being developed. Like CEM, nuclear imaging of the breast provides an alternative functional imaging tool for those patients unable to undergo breast MRI.[23]

- Abbreviated breast MRI (AB-MRI):

AB-MRI protocols seek to reduce time and cost of performing and interpreting breast magnetic resonance (MR) studies in a screening setting via a precontrast and single early postcontrast T1-weighted series that can be obtained in less than 10 to 15 minutes. Standard breast MRI scan time is approximately 30 to 45 minutes and can be difficult to tolerate, particularly for claustrophobic patients. Reducing the time and cost of breast MR screening can improve access to breast MR screening for a wider population, providing superior sensitivity for cancer detection than either ultrasonography or tomosynthesis.[24]

- Computed tomography of the breast

Breast computed tomography provides true isotropic 3D imaging of the breasts without the need for breast compression. Imaging is obtained after the intravenous administration of iodinated contrast material, so both anatomic and physiologic information is provided. Although the technology is still under investigation, data have been promising thus far in the diagnostic setting. Radiation dose remains one of the greatest

Table 2
Pros and cons of each imaging modality

	Pros	Cons
Digital mammography, 2D	• Cost effective • Widely available • Sensitive • Has proven mortality benefit	Lower sensitivity in dense breasts
DBT	• Sensitive • Slightly higher cancer detection rate than 2D mammography • Fewer recalls than 2D mammography	Lower sensitivity in extremely dense breasts
Breast ultrasonography	• Relatively high sensitivity and specificity • Can distinguish cystic from solid lesions • Can facilitate best-tolerated image-guided biopsy • Can be performed safely at any age as there is no ionizing radiation	Operator dependent Targeted ultrasonography requires specific requisition to improve accuracy
Breast MRI	• Highly sensitive • Most accurately documents disease extent	Variable but generally lower specificity Expensive Not tolerated by all patients Less widely available so awaiting MRI can delay treatment

challenges, with work ongoing to reduce the dose; this may provide another similar but less costly alternative to breast MRI.[25]

A NOTE OF CAUTION

Thermography: Thermography involves creating a temperature map of the breasts on the basis of infrared radiation, with the hypothesis that breast cancers exhibit higher temperatures due to higher metabolism and angiogenesis relative to that of normal breast. Thermography ultimately proved to be insensitive as a screening modality and provides no added benefit over mammography alone.

Mammographic Findings

A radiologist interprets and reports mammography results using the BI-RADS, published by the American College of Radiology. BI-RADS was originally devised in the 1980s with the purpose of creating a system for standardized reporting of mammography studies to address prior ambiguity in communication of findings and recommendations to the referring clinician.[26–28]

BI-RADS uses an assessment scale from 0 through 6 to indicate a final assessment of the mammogram (**Table 3**) as well as recommendations to the referring physician.

In the BI-RADS report, the radiologist also includes a score for breast density on a scale from A through D:

A. *Almost entirely fatty (10% of women)*: The breasts are composed almost entirely of fatty tissue and contain very little fibrous and glandular tissue.
B. *Scattered areas of fibroglandular density (40% of women)*: The breasts are mostly fatty tissue, but there are a few areas of fibrous and glandular tissue visible on the mammogram.
C. *Heterogeneously dense (40% of women)*: A mammogram shows many areas of fibrous and glandular tissue or a large amount of tissue in a single area.
D. *Extremely dense (10% of women)*: The breasts have large amounts of fibrous and glandular tissue.

Women with dense breasts are more likely to

- be premenopausal
- use postmenopausal hormone replacement therapy
- have a lower body mass index

When interpreting a mammogram, the radiologist will note the presence or absence of one or more of the following radiographic lesions (findings) and provide a recommendation to the clinician. If a biopsy is recommended and then performed, the radiologist will issue an addendum to the biopsy report indicating further recommendations based on diagnosis and concordance.

The most commonly reported imaging findings are as follows.

Masses

Benign features: oval shape, circumscribed margins, low density, or fat containing.

Suspicious features: round or irregular shape, microlobulated, indistinct or speculated margins, high density.

Asymmetries

Asymmetry: one-view mammographic finding most commonly a summation artifact

Focal asymmetry: 2-view mammographic finding occupying less than 1 quadrant that is not clearly a mass.

Global asymmetry: relative to the contralateral breast, represents a large area of fibroglandular tissue involving at least one quadrant, usually benign.

Developing asymmetry: focal asymmetry that is new, larger, or more conspicuous than on prior examination, about 15% are malignant.

Architectural distortion. Parenchyma appears distorted without a definite mass; this can be postsurgical or posttraumatic but is otherwise suspicious for malignancy or radial scar and tissue diagnosis is appropriate.

Calcifications: Best Evaluated with Magnification Images. Benign features: dermal, vascular, coarse or popcornlike, large rodlike, round, rim, dystrophic, milk of calcium (layering), suture, diffuse, regional.

Suspicious features: amorphous, coarse heterogeneous, fine pleomorphic, fine linear branching, grouped, linear, segmental.

It is important to note the substantial overlap in the imaging appearance of benign and malignant entities. For this reason, lesions are managed based on their most concerning imaging feature and image-guided biopsy is recommended even for many lesions with largely benign imaging features. Any finding with a greater than 2% likelihood of malignancy is appropriate for biopsy.

Table 3	
BI-RADS assessment	
BI-RADS Assessment	**Management**
BI-RADS 0: Incomplete: Need additional imaging evaluation and/or prior mammographies for comparison	Recall for additional imaging and/or comparison with prior examinations
BI-RADS 1: Negative	Routine mammography screening
BI-RADS 2: Benign	Routine mammography screening
BI-RADS 3: Probably benign	Short-interval follow-up
BI-RADS 4: Suspicious	Tissue diagnosis
BI-RADS 5: Highly suspicious	Tissue diagnosis
BI-RADS 6: Known biopsy-proven malignancy	Surgical excision when clinically appropriate

Image-guided percutaneous biopsy

Why Percutaneous Biopsy and Not Surgical Biopsy

Percutaneous biopsy of breast lesions is considered standard of care and a quality metric for health care facilities. The patient-related advantages of percutaneous breast biopsy include diminished invasiveness compared with surgery, less scarring, and minimal delay. Complication rates are extremely low, and surgical planning is optimized.[29]

Image-guided biopsy can be performed using mammographic guidance (known as a stereotactic or tomosynthesis-guided biopsy), sonographic guidance, or MRI guidance. When possible, biopsies are performed under ultrasound guidance because this optimizes patient comfort and is generally the fastest technique. Biopsies performed under ultrasound guidance include fine-needle aspirations (FNAs) and core needle biopsies. In a core needle biopsy, a needle typically ranging in size from 18 to 9 gauge is advanced into the target and a core of tissue removed. Several samples are obtained and sent in formalin for pathologic review. In an FNA, a small needle (typically 18–25 gauge) is moved rapidly back and forth within the targeted lesion to obtain cells for diagnosis. The cells are examined by a cytopathologist who first determines whether they are sufficient for diagnosis and then provides an assessment. Although the presence or absence of malignant cells can be determined in most cases, the structural information available in a core needle biopsy specimen is lost and therefore the pathologic diagnosis provided can usually be less specific.

Stereotactic biopsies are generally reserved for those findings that are not sonographically apparent, most commonly calcifications. A core needle (typically 9 gauge) is advanced to the target calculated by the machine, and several core samples are obtained. An MRI-guided biopsy is similarly performed in an MRI machine following the administration of intravenous contrast. Both techniques are typically more time consuming than ultrasound-guided biopsies but are important in evaluating lesions that are not sonographically evident.

The placement of a specially designed biopsy marker clip is essential following nearly all imaging-guided biopsies. This clip enables accurate localization of the biopsied area before surgery. If surgery is not required, the clip serves as an important indication on follow-up imaging that the area has undergone prior biopsy. Biopsy marker clips are also often key to confirming correlation of imaging findings on multiple modalities. Most currently available clips are made of titanium, stainless steel, or a nickel-containing compound. Clips are MRI compatible and extremely safe. The incidence of allergic reaction is extremely low.[30]

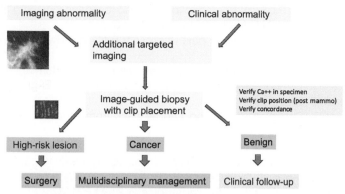

Fig. 1. Management of radiographic breast lesions.

Following an image-guided biopsy, a 2-view postbiopsy mammography is typically performed to document clip placement and, in many cases, confirm correlation of the imaging findings on different modalities. This mammogram can also help with planning if a needle localization procedure is needed. When pathology results are available, an assessment of radiographic-pathologic correlation is essential; if the pathologic results are discordant with the imaging findings, repeat sampling of the area must be performed by repeat percutaneous biopsy or surgery. A graphic depiction of the management of radiologic breast lesions is shown in **Fig. 1**.

SUMMARY

High-quality breast imaging, communication with the radiologist, and thoughtful review of biopsy results are essential steps in everyday breast surgical oncology practice. An understanding of an imaging modality and its interpretation improve quality of care and efficiency in managing patients. In an effort to minimize radiation exposure, inappropriate testing, and misdiagnosis, a clear understanding of the role of each imaging study as it relates to the individual patients is key.

CLINICS CARE POINTS

- High-quality breast imaging and interpretation are essential for complete evaluation of the patient with breast cancer
- Mammography, ultrasonography, and in selective cases MRI represent the cornerstones of diagnostic breast imaging
- Image-guided percutaneous needle biopsy is the optimal means of tissue sampling when this is recommended

DISCLOSURE

The authors have nothing to disclose.

REFERENCES

1. Strax P, Venet L, Shapiro S. Value of mammography in reduction of mortality from breast cancer in mass screening. Am J Roentgenol Radium Ther Nucl Med 1973; 117(3):686–9.

2. Scatliff JH, Morris PJ. From Roentgen to magnetic resonance imaging: the history of medical imaging. N C Med J 2014;75(2):111–3.

3. The evolution of breast imaging: past to present B N joe. Edward Sickles Radiol 2014;273(2).

4. Pisano ED, Gatsonis C, Hendrick E, et al. Diagnostic performance of digital versus film mammography for breast-cancer screening. N Engl J Med 2005; 353(17):1773–83.

5. Hendrick RE. Radiation doses and cancer risks from breast imaging studies. Radiology 2010;257(1):246–53.

6. Dershaw DD, Fleischman RC, Liberman L, et al. Use of digital mammography in needle localization procedures. AJR Am J Roentgenol 1993;161(3):559–62.

7. Gao Y, Moy L, Heller S. Digital breast tomosynthesis: update on technology, evidence, and clinical practice. Radiographics 2021;41:321–37.

8. Chong A, Weinstein SP, McDonald ES, et al. Digital breast tomosynthesis: concepts and clinical practice. Radiology 2019;292:1–14.

9. Taylor KJ, Merritt C, Piccoli C, et al. Ultrasound as a complement to mammography and breast examination to characterize breast masses. Ultrasound Med Biol 2002;28(1):19–26.

10. Berg WA, Blume JD, Cormack JB, et al. Combined screening with ultrasound and mammography vs mammography alone in women at elevated risk of breast cancer. JAMA 2008;299(18):2151–63.

11. Berg WA, Blume JD, Cormack JB, et al. Operator dependence of physician-performed whole-breast US: lesion detection and characterization. Radiology 2006;241(2):355–65.

12. Price ER, Hargreaves J, Lipson JA, et al. The California breast density information group: a collaborative response to the issues of breast density, breast cancer risk, and breast density notification legislation. Radiology 2013;269(3):887–92.

13. Butler RS, Hooley RJ. Screening breast ultrasound:update after 10 years of breast density notification laws. AJR 2020;214:1424–35.

14. Kolb TM, Lichy J, Newhouse JH. Comparison of the performance of screening mammography, physical examination, and breast US and evaluation of factors that influence them: An analysis of 27,825 patient evaluations. Radiology 2002; 225:165–75.

15. Berg WA, Zhang Z, Lehrer D, et al. Detection of breast cancer with addition of annual screening ultrasound or a single screening MRI to mammography in women with elevated breast cancer risk. JAMA 2012;307:1394–404.

16. Harvey JA, Yaffe MJ, D'Orsi C, et al. Density and breast cancer risk. Radiology 2013;267(2):657–8.

17. Yi A, Jang M, Yim D, et al. Addition of screening breast US to digital mammography and digital breast tomosynthesis for breast cancer screening in women at average risk. Radiology 2021;298:568–75.

18. Lee CH, Dershaw DD, Kopans D, et al. Breast cancer screening with imaging: recommendations from the Society of Breast Imaging and the ACR on the use of mammography, breast MRI, breast ultrasound, and other technologies for the detection of clinically occult breast cancer. J Am Coll Radiol 2010;7(1):18–27.

19. Raber B, Bea VJ, Bedrosian I. How Does MR Imaging Help Care for My Breast Cancer Patient? Perspective of a Surgical Oncologist. Magn Reson Imaging Clin N Am 2018;26(2):281–8.

20. Reig B, Lewin AA, Du L, et al. Breast MRI for Evaluation of Response to Neoadjuvant Therapy. Radiographics 2021;41(3):665–79.

21. Brenner RJ. Evaluation of breast silicone implants. Magn Reson Imaging Clin N Am 2013;21(3):547–60.
22. Jochelson MS, Lobbes MBI. Contrast-enhanced mammography: state of the art. Radiology 2021;299:36–48.
23. Berg WA. Nuclear breast imaging: clinical results and future directions. JNM 2016;57:46S–52S.
24. Kuhl CK, Schrading S, Strobel K, et al. Abbreviated breast magnetic resonance imaging (MRI): first postcontrast subtracted images and maximum-intensity projection-a novel approach to breast cancer screening with MRI. J Clin Oncol 2014; 32(22):2304–10.
25. Zhu Y, O'Connell AM, Yue M, et al. Dedicated breast CT: state of the art—part I. Historical evolution and technical aspects. Eur Radiol 2022;32:1579–89.
26. Kopans DB. Standardized mammography reporting. Radiol Clin North Am 1992; 30(1):257–64.
27. Burnside ES, Sickles EA, Bassett LW, et al. The ACR BI-RADS experience: learning from history. J Am Coll Radiol 2009;6(12):851–60, 51.
28. Sickles EA. Periodic mam) [ACR BI-RADS® atlas, breast imaging reporting and data system. Reston (VA): American College of Radiology; 2013.
29. Liberman L. Centennial dissertation. Percutaneous imaging-guided core breast biopsy: state of the art at the millennium. AJR Am J Roentgenol 2000;174(5): 1191–9.
30. Portnow LH, Thornton CM, Milch HS, et al. Biopsy marker standardization: what's in a name? AJR 2019;212:1400–5.

Dermatological Conditions of the Breast

Srinidhi Pulusani, MD[a], Emily Jones, MD[a], Alyssa D. Throckmorton, MD[b,c],*

KEYWORDS

- Dermatology of breast skin • Nipple • And areola

KEY POINTS

- Most skin findings on the breast do not represent breast cancer.
- Infectious conditions are often fungal or viral in nature.
- Atopic, allergic, and irritant dermatitis can be treated with removal of the offending agent, emollients, topical steroids, with phototherapy and systemic medications for recalcitrant cases.

INTRODUCTION

Many visits to a breast specialist involve concerns related to the skin of the breast, not the breast parenchyma itself. There are a wide variety of skin disorders that can present on the skin of the breast, chest, and axilla ranging from malignancies to infections to inflammatory conditions. Some of these may present during breastfeeding. Often these are directed to the breast surgeon for concern of inflammatory breast cancer or Paget's disease or because they are thought to require surgery for management, such as hidradenitis.

A thorough history and physical are indicated including past medical history, autoimmune diseases in the patient or family, family cancer history, medications, immunization status, breast imaging, breast examination, and examination of the skin on other parts of the body. Questions should be asked regarding initial symptoms, changes or duration of skin lesions, prior episodes, alleviating or aggravating factors, and any changes in medications or substances contacting the skin.

This review was designed as a dermatology primer for breast surgeons to include the most common neoplasms (**Table 1**), infectious processes and their mimickers (**Table 2**), and inflammatory conditions (**Table 3**) that can present on or involve the breast.

[a] Department of Dermatology, University of Tennessee Health Science Center, 930 Madison Avenue, Suite 840, Memphis, TN 38163, USA; [b] Department of Surgery, University of Tennessee Health Science Center, Memphis, TN, USA; [c] Breast Program, Baptist Medical Group, 7205 Wolf River Boulevard, Suite 200, Germantown, TN 38138, USA
* Corresponding author. 7205 Wolf River Boulevard, Suite 200, Germantown, TN 38138.
E-mail address: alyssa.throckmorton@bmg.md
Twitter: @throckad (A.D.T.)

Surg Clin N Am 102 (2022) 1043–1063
https://doi.org/10.1016/j.suc.2022.07.003
surgical.theclinics.com
0039-6109/22/© 2022 Elsevier Inc. All rights reserved.

Table 1
Neoplasm summary

Neoplasm	Breast Location	Other Common Locations	Painful	Pruritic	Appearance	Risk Factors	Biopsy Needed/Helpful
Paget's	Unilateral nipple	None	No	No	Scaly or ulcerated nipple	Usual breast cancer risk factors	Yes
Inflammatory breast cancer	Any	None	Yes	Maybe	Erythematous skin, skin edema (Peau d' orange)	Same as breast cancer risk factors	Maybe
Dermatofibrosarcoma protuberans	Any	Trunk, proximal extremities, head, neck	No	No	Slow growing, small, firm, skin-colored plaque or raised lesion	Young to middle age, women, Blacks	Yes
Cutaneous T cell Lymphoma	Any	Buttocks, thighs, chest, abdomen, back	No	No	Erythematous scaly patches, telangiectasia, mottled hypo or hyperpigmentation		Yes
Basal cell Cancer	Upper chest	Face, head, neck, arms legs	No	No	Flesh colored pearl or pink patch	Lifetime sun exposure, immunosuppression	Yes
Squamous cell cancer	Upper chest	Face, ears, neck, back, arms	No	No	Red, firm, raised lesions or scaly patches	Lifetime sun exposure, pale lighter skin, immunosuppression	Yes
Melanoma	Any	Any skin, mucosal surfaces, retina, meninges, dura, eye	No	No	Darkly pigmented lesions with irregular borders, multiple colors	Sun exposure, tanning bed, men, prior skin cancer, family history, immunosuppression	Yes
Seborrheic keratoses	Any	Any	No	No	Tan to brown, papillomatous, papules or plaques	Older age	No

Table 2
Infections and their mimickers

Infectious Conditions and Mimickers	Breast Location	Other Common Locations	Painful	Pruritic	Appearance	Risk Factors	Biopsy Needed/Helpful
Tinea Corporis	any	any	No	Yes	Annular scaly plaques	immunosuppression	No (KOH can help)
Tinea Versicolor	Central chest	Upper back, shoulders	No	Yes	Hyper- or hypopigmented thin scaly macules	Worse in hot climate, summer months	No (KOH can help)
Candidiasis	Infra-mammary	Mucocutaneous sites, lower abdomen	No	Yes	Erythematous plaque with satellite pustules	Obesity, immunosuppression	No
Herpes Zoster	Dermatomal	Face, back	Yes	No	Clustered vesicles on an erythematous base	Older age, immunosuppression	No
Hidradenitis Suppurativa	Infra-mammary	Axillae, inguinal folds, gluteal cleft	Yes	No	Nodules and tracts with purulent drainage	Female, African American	No
Pyoderma Gangrenosum	Any	Any	Yes	No	Deep ulcer with overhanging gray border	IBD, RA	Yes (rule out other causes)

Table 3
Inflammatory condition summary

Inflammatory Conditions	Breast Location	Other Common Locations	Painful	Pruritic	Appearance	Risk Factors	Biopsy Needed/Helpful
Atopic dermatitis	Usually nipple	Any	No	Yes	Erythematous scaly papules and plaques	Genetic and environmental factors	No
Contact dermatitis	Any	Any	No	Yes	Pruritic, erythematous, edematous papules and plaques	Eczema	No
Seborrheic dermatitis	Central chest	Scalp, face, ears	No	Yes	Erythematous patches with greasy scale	Host response to Malassezia, Parkinson's disease	No
CARP	Central chest	Neck, back	No	Mild	Brown keratotic verrucous papules and reticulated plaques	Endocrine imbalance, host response to Malassezia	No
Benign familial pemphigus	Inframammary	Intertriginous (axillae, inguinal folds)	Yes	No	Flaccid blisters and erosions, foul-smelling vegetative plaques	Autosomal dominant	Maybe
Psoriasis	Any	Usually scalp, elbows, lower back, knees	No	Yes	Erythematous patches and thin plaques with or without white scale	Family history, environmental factors, preceding streptococcal infection	Maybe
Morphea	Any	Any	Maybe	No	Erythematous or violaceous plaques that progress to atrophic plaques with a violaceous border	Mechanical trauma, radiation, injections	Yes
Lichen sclerosus	Any	Genitalia, chest, upper back, abdomen	Maybe	Maybe	Blueish-white papules and plaques that process to atrophic plaques with telangiectasias	HLA-DQ7 autoantibodies, antibodies to ECM-1, concomitant autoimmune disease (thyroid disease, vitiligo)	Yes

Condition							
Hyperkeratosis of the nipple & areola	Nipple, areola	None	No	Mild	Hyperpigmented verrucous papules and plaques	May be hormonally driven	No
Cyst of Montgomery	Areola	None	No	No	Erythematous nodule if inflamed or obstructed	none	No
Radiation dermatitis	Any	Any	Maybe	Maybe	Variable: mild erythema, ulceration, necrosis	Prior radiation therapy	Yes
Pemphigus	Any	Any	Yes	No	Crusted erythematous erosions	Can be associated with malignancy	Yes
Raynaud's	Nipple	Fingers, toes	Yes	No	Nipple discoloration	Cold climate, nicotine use, family history, systemic sclerosis	No
Superficial thrombophlebitis	Any	Chest wall	Yes	No	Erythematous, tender, linear cord	Recent surgery, hormone therapy, infection, tight clothing	No
Calciphylaxis	Any	Any	Yes	No	Ulcerated, necrotic plaques	End-stage renal disease, warfarin use	Yes

NEOPLASMS
Seborrheic Keratosis

Seborrheic keratoses (SKs) are benign growths that develop in men and women during adulthood. The pathogenesis of SKs is thought to be multifactorial and may be related to the disruption of epidermal growth factor receptors. SKs present as tan to dark brown papillomatous, waxy papules, and small plaques on the trunk, face, or extremities. The "stuck on" appearance with or without an overlying scale can help differentiate SKs from melanoma.[1] SKs are commonly asymptomatic; although, they can become inflamed or pruritic. Typically, the onset of SKs is gradual over years. A sudden eruption of SKs, referred to as the "Leser-Trelat sign" can be associated with multiple malignancies, including breast cancer.[2] Due to the benign nature of SKs, the lesions can be monitored or excised if symptomatic or located in cosmetically sensitive areas.

Paget's Disease

Paget's disease is a rare presentation of breast cancer. The skin of the nipple can present with eczematous type findings, ulceration, or erosion with unilateral involvement. Clinical findings may be confined to the skin but in more than 90% of cases, the underlying breast parenchyma is involved with invasive breast cancer or at least, ductal carcinoma in situ.[3] Treatment is similar to other early-stage breast cancers and may be driven by the extent of the underlying breast involvement.

Inflammatory Breast Cancer

Inflammatory breast cancer represents 2% of all breast cancers. There are no current molecular markers to distinguish inflammatory from noninflammatory breast cancer and therefore, is considered a clinical diagnosis. Patients with inflammatory breast cancers present with rapidly evolving skin changes including diffuse erythema and induration.[4] National Comprehensive Cancer Network (NCCN) guidelines require erythema and edema of at least one-third of the breast for a clinical diagnosis of inflammatory breast cancer.[5] Skin punch biopsy can confirm the diagnosis if dermal lymphatic involvement is identified histologically but a negative result does not exclude inflammatory breast cancer.[4] An expert panel recommended using a time interval to distinguish between true inflammatory breast cancer ($</ = 6$ months) and one with secondary erythema from locally advanced breast cancer (6 months).[6] Most inflammatory breast cancers present with regional nodal involvement, and many will also present with distant metastases.[4] A multimodal treatment approach including chemotherapy, surgery and radiation are used when treating for curative intent.

Dermatofibrosarcoma Protuberans

Dermatofibrosarcoma protuberans (DSFP) are a rare, low-grade malignancy originating from the fibroblastic mesenchymal cells in the dermis. It represents less than 0.1% of all malignancies. The most common locations to find a DSFP are the trunk (40%–50%), proximal extremities (30%–40%), head, and neck (10%–15%). The incidence is higher in women and Black patients, and the highest incidence is between ages 25 to 45. DSFPs have been reported in patients with immunodeficiency conditions as well as pregnancy.[7] Infrequently, these can be found in the breast.[8] In the early stages, these present as a slow-growing, painless, firm, skin-colored plaque, or protuberance. Biopsy is recommended for diagnosis. Surgical excision with wide local excision or Mohs micrographic surgery can be used depending on the location involved. DSFP involving the trunk are commonly treated with wide local excision.

NCCN guidelines recommend a 2–4 cm margin.[9] Adjuvant radiation may be considered for fibrosarcomatous variant or if excision for DSFP did not achieve at least 1 cm margins.[7]

Dermatologic Malignancies

For squamous cell carcinoma (SCC), basal cell carcinoma (BCC) and melanoma, ultraviolet (UV) solar radiation is the main factor in development. UV exposure induces carcinogenesis through DNA damage causing mutations as well as the decreased ability of the immune system to recognize and remove these malignant cells. Cumulative UV exposure is directly related to the risk of developing SCC and BCC while sun exposure specifically during adolescence is the main risk for melanoma. There are other risk factors including family history, chemical exposure, use of tanning beds, human papillomavirus, skin type, presence of melanocytic nevi, and immunosuppression, such as in organ transplant recipients.[10]

Basal Cell Carcinoma

These are the least aggressive skin cancers. These present as a flesh-colored pearly or pink patch of skin. Given the pathogenesis, these are mostly found on the sun-exposed skin, such as the face, head, neck, arms, legs, and abdomen. It is rare but BCC has been reported on the nipple and areolar complex (NAC) with a higher rate of metastasis, 9.1%.[11,12] When BCC occurs on the NAC, it is more likely in men as this area has less sun exposure in women. These are diagnosed with a skin biopsy and can be treated with topical 5-fluorouracil if superficial.[13] Surgical excision is an option but patients who are poor operative candidates, but have aggressive or recurrent forms, may be treated with radiation or systemic medication.[10]

Squamous Cell Carcinoma

Squamous cell carcinomas form from the keratinocytes in the epidermis. These can be seen as red, firm bumps or scaly patches in sun-exposed skin, most commonly ear, face, neck, chest, and back. Ulceration can develop if untreated. They are more common in patients with pale, lighter skin.[13] These are diagnosed by skin biopsy. Treatment can include photodynamic therapy, topical chemotherapy agents, curettage, and electrodessication or surgical excision.[10]

Melanoma

Melanoma represents a small percentage of skin cancers but is considered more deadly than other skin cancers. The overall incidence is rising. Melanomas arise from the uncontrolled growth and proliferation of melanocytes. These are usually found in the dermis of the skin but can arise anywhere melanocytes are found.[14] Approximately 4% to 5% of melanomas are found in noncutaneous sites such as mucosal surfaces, the eye, dura, or meninges. There are cases reports of primary melanoma of the breast itself.[15] These often present as pigmented lesions with asymmetrical lesions, irregular borders, uneven coloring, size greater than 0.4 cm, or evolving lesions (**Fig. 1**). Early-stage cutaneous melanomas are treated with surgical excision with margin width and sentinel node surgery depending on the thickness of the melanoma. Later stage disease can now also be treated with adjuvant targeted therapies and immune checkpoint inhibitors.[16]

INFECTIONS
Fungal Infections

Tinea corporis appears as annular scaly plaques on the trunk or extremities caused by a dermatophyte infection limited to the stratum corneum. Tinea versicolor can appear

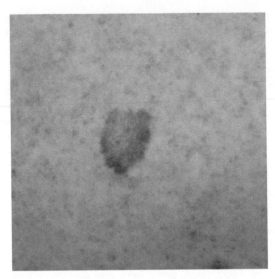

Fig. 1. Melanoma.

as hyper- or hypopigmented small round patches with fine scale, favoring seborrheic areas such as the central chest but can extend onto the breast. Scale becoming more apparent after scraping or stretching the skin is called the evoked scale sign and can help differentiate from other conditions.[17,18] Residual pigmentary alteration can often take weeks to months to improve, but does not signal treatment failure, and patients should be counseled accordingly. Mucocutaneous candidiasis is common in the inframammary folds and presents as erythematous patches often with satellite papules and pustules. Diagnosis, causative organisms, and treatment are in **Table 4**.[18]

Herpes Zoster (shingles)

Herpes zoster is due to the reactivation of varicella zoster virus. It is characterized by a painful eruption of clustered vesicles which is usually preceded by pain in the affected area. It erupts in a dermatomal distribution and can involve the breast when involving dermatomes T1–T5. Diagnosis is usually made by clinical appearance alone, but can be confirmed with Tzanck smear, PCR, DFA, or viral culture. Acyclovir, valacyclovir, and famciclovir are FDA approved for treating herpes zoster and one of these options should be initiated as soon as possible during the disease course to prevent postherpetic neuralgia. Patients with moderate to severe pain from herpes zoster can be started on gabapentin or low-dose tricyclic antidepressants to prevent postherpetic neuralgia.[19]

INFLAMMATORY
Hidradenitis Suppurativa

Hidradenitis Suppurative (HS) is a chronic inflammatory skin disease primarily affecting the intertriginous or apocrine gland-bearing areas, including axillae (**Fig. 2**), breast (**Fig. 3**), and groin.[20] HS affects about 1% of the population and is more common in women and Black patients.[21] Characteristic skin lesions of HS include double comedones, nodules, abscesses, and sinus tracks which lead to scarring.[22] HS is graded using the Hurley scale. Obesity, smoking, polycystic ovarian syndrome, and metabolic syndrome are associated with HS, and HS can lead to decreased quality

Table 4
Summary for fungal infections[19]

Diagnosis	Causative Organism	Diagnosis	Treatment
Tinea versicolor	Malassezia (Pityrosporum) yeasts	KOH examination of skin scrapings with both hyphal and yeast forms; "spaghetti and meatballs"	*Topical ketoconazole shampoo or cream* Alternatives: zinc pyrithione and selenium-containing shampoos used as a body wash
Tinea corporis	Microsporum, Trichophyton, and Epidermophyton species	KOH examination of a skin scraping showing branching hyphae	*Topical terbinafine cream or topical azole creams (clotrimazole, econazole)* Alternatives: May consider oral antifungals (terbinafine, griseofulvin, azole antifungals) if recalcitrant to topical therapy
Candida	C. Albicans	Usually by the clinical appearance. Can do fungal culture or KOH scraping showing budding yeast and pseudohyphae	*Topical nystatin cream or topical azole (ketoconazole) antifungals* Alternatives: May consider oral fluconazole if recalcitrant to topical therapy

of life and depression.[21] The exact pathophysiology of HS remains unknown, but current research suggest it is hyperkeratosis and rupture of the follicular unit, followed by the upregulation of autoinflammatory pathways.[23] Treatment options are outlined in **Table 5**[20]

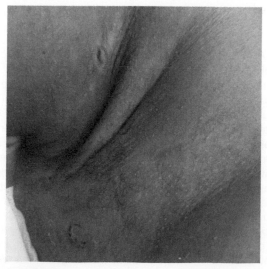

Fig. 2. Axillary hidradenitis.

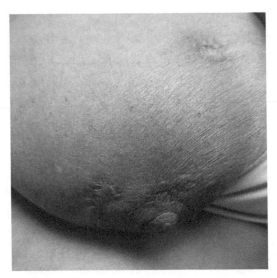

Fig. 3. Hidradenitis on the breast.

Pyoderma Gangrenosum

Pyoderma gangrenosum (PG) is a rare neutrophilic dermatosis characterized by rapidly progressive, painful ulceration (**Fig. 4**). It occurs most commonly on the lower limbs, but can occur on the breast, especially after biopsy or surgery due to a process termed pathergy.[24] It can often be misdiagnosed as a wound infection after surgery and should be considered in cases whereby standard therapy is unsuccessful.[24] Clinically, PG begins as an inflammatory papule or pustule that expands into an exudative painful ulcer with gray overhanging borders.[25,26] Other underlying conditions associated with PG include inflammatory bowel disease and rheumatoid arthritis.[26] Management includes immunosuppressant therapy such as oral corticosteroids and TNF-alpha inhibitors, avoiding surgical debridement, and applying nonadherent dressings.[25]

Atopic Dermatitis

Atopic dermatitis (AD) is an inflammatory condition affecting 10% to 30% of children and 2% to 10% of adults. AD is caused by both genetic and environmental factors leading to epidermal barrier dysfunction, immune dysregulation, and alterations of the cutaneous microbiome.[27] AD is characterized by a broad clinical spectrum. In adolescents and adults, lichenified plaques with variable amounts of scale, crust, and fissuring are typically seen. Nipple eczema is a common presentation of AD in women (**Fig. 5**). It is typically bilateral and primarily seen in adolescent girls but can also present during pregnancy and breastfeeding.[22,28] When seen in breastfeeding, it can predispose lactating women to bacterial or viral super-infection.[27] Nipple eczema can be exacerbated by chronic friction and can be seen in runners or other athletes. AD on the breast can be managed like presentation elsewhere on the body; however, care should be taken to minimize the use of super potent topical steroids as the breast tissue is thin and prone to atrophy. First-line treatments include low-moderate potency topical steroids, calcipotriene cream, and topical calcineurin inhibitors. Special consideration should be taken when treating lactating women as all medications cannot safely be consumed. Patients should be instructed to wipe off any topical

Table 5
Hidradenitis treatment by Hurley stage[20,24]

Hurley Stage	Topical Medical Therapy	Systemic Medical Therapy	Surgical Treatment

I	Clindamycin 1%
	Resorcinol 12%
	Benzoyl peroxide 5 or 10%
	Antimicrobial washes:
	Benzoyl peroxide or chlorhexidine
		Doxycycline 100 mg twice daily
		Adjunctive hormonal therapy:
		    Oral contraceptives
		    ± spironolactone
			• Intralesional triamcinolone (3–5 mg), repeat monthly as needed
			• May consider punch debridement or excision of individual lesions

II	See above	First line: Doxycycline 100 mg (or other tetracycline antibiotics) twice daily Second line: Clindamycin 300 mg twice daily- monotherapy OR Clindamycin-Rifampin combination • Clindamycin 300 mg twice daily • Rifampin 300 mg twice daily Third line: TNF-α inhibitors • Adalimumab 40 mg q wk (after loading dose)	Intralesion triamcinolone (see above) May consider punch debridement or excision of individual lesions Deroofing of sinus tracts Sinus tract excisions Carbon dioxide laser
III	See above	See above for first and second line Third line: TNF-α inhibitors Adalimumab 40 mg q wk (after loading dose) OR Infliximab 5 mg/kg every 8 wk (after loading dose)	See above Radical wide local excision

Data from Saunte DML, Jemec GBE. Hidradenitis Suppurativa: Advances in Diagnosis and Treatment. JAMA. Nov 28 2017;318(20):2019-2032. https://doi.org/10.1001/jama.2017.16691 and Orenstein LAV, Nguyen TV, Damiani G, Sayed C, Jemec GBE, Hamzavi I. Medical and Surgical Management of Hidradenitis Suppurativa: A Review of International Treatment Guidelines and Implementation in General Dermatology Practice. Dermatology. 2020;236(5):393-412. https://doi.org/10.1159/000507323.

medications before breastfeeding.[22] While many patients are able to achieve adequate control with topical therapies and emollient use, patients with recalcitrant AD may require phototherapy or systemic medications, including Dupilumab.[29,30]

Contact Dermatitis

Contact dermatitis can be divided based on the causative agent, either allergic or irritant. Allergic contact dermatitis (ACD) is caused by a type 4 delayed hypersensitivity reaction.[31] ACD acutely presents as pruritic, erythematous, edematous papules and plaques, which commonly can be weeping or blistering (**Fig. 6**). Chronically, well-demarcated lichenified scaly plaques are seen in the affected areas. Common allergens involved in ACD on the breast include Cl + Me-isothiazolinone, a preservative seen in detergents, sanitary wipes, and fabric softeners, cobalt chloride, seen in metal

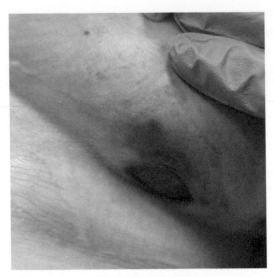

Fig. 4. Pyoderma gangrenosum.

fasteners and jewelry, and nickel sulfate, also seen in metal fasteners.[32] Cyanoacrylate glue, commonly known as Dermabond, has also been shown to cause ACD when used for wound closure. Cross-reaction with other acrylate products, such as cosmetic products including acrylic nails and eyelash extension glue, can trigger a delayed-type hypersensitivity response with Dermabond use.[33]

The management of ACD is centered around the identification of causative allergen, patient education, and treatment of symptoms. Patch testing can be performed to determine the causative agent. Once identified, extreme care should be taken to avoid the allergen. Skin inflammation can be treated, with topical steroids and moisturization.[31] Irritant contact dermatitis (ICD) is a nonimmunological phenomenon caused by the direct cytotoxic effect due to a chemical or physical insult. Clinical findings

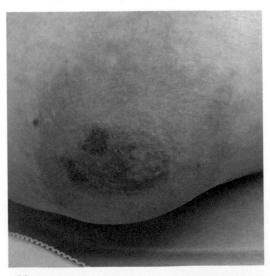

Fig. 5. Nipple dermatitis or eczema.

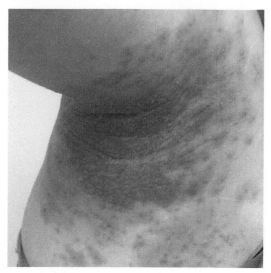

Fig. 6. Allergic contact dermatitis.

are typically well-demarcated, polymorphic, and can include erythema, edema, ulcerations, and necrosis. On the breast, ICD can result from exercise, mechanical injury, or moisture-related injury during breastfeeding.[22,34]

Seborrheic Dermatitis

Seborrheic dermatitis is an inflammatory condition found in infants, children, and adults. In adults, seborrheic dermatitis is chronic and is mostly seen in the 5th and 6th decades of life. Seborrheic dermatitis occurs in areas of active sebaceous glands, such as the scalp, glabellar area, nasolabial folds, and central chest. Seborrheic dermatitis is typically found on the central chest rather than the inframammary folds, as seen in intertrigo. It is thought to be triggered by a commensal yeast, *Malassezia furfur*, which has been isolated from cutaneous sebaceous glands. Clinical findings of seborrheic dermatitis include erythematous patches with the overly greasy scale with or without vesiculation and crust.[35] The management of seborrheic dermatitis is targeted at controlling levels of Malassezia with topical azole shampoos or creams and controlling inflammation with low-potency topical steroids. Patients should also be counseled that seborrheic dermatitis is a chronic condition and maintenance treatment should be used to avoid flares.[35]

Confluent and Reticulated Papillomatosis

Confluent and reticulated papillomatosis (CARP) is a benign proliferation seen in teenagers and young adults. CARP is more common in female patients. The etiology of CARP is unclear and may be related to endocrine imbalance, dysfunctional keratinization, or host response to *M furfur*. The clinical presentation consists of asymptotic or mildly pruritic brown keratotic, verrucous papules that coalescence in a thin reticulated plaque on the intermammary area (**Fig. 7**), neck, and back (**Fig. 8**).[1] CARP can be treated with oral tetracyclines, topical antifungals, or combination therapies.[36]

Psoriasis

Psoriasis is a chronic inflammatory disorder resulting from genetic predisposition and environmental triggers. Onset is bimodal with peaks between 20 and 30 years of age

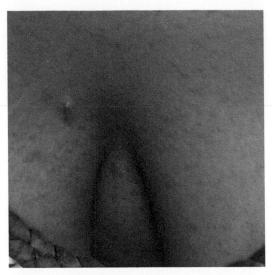

Fig. 7. CARP presenting in the intramammary region

and 50 and 60 years of age. Patients will often report a positive family history of psoriasis. Pathogenesis of disease is thought to be related to the increased activity of T-helper cells and numerous cytokines. In genetically predisposed patients, triggers such as the Koebner phenomenon (onset after injury to the skin), infections, stress, and certain medication use can elicit the onset of psoriatic disease.[37]

Any area of the breast and nipple can be involved but when the inframammary fold, as well as other intertriginous areas, are involved, it is termed inverse psoriasis (**Fig. 9**). Inverse psoriasis can be mistaken for intertrigo, candida infection, or seborrheic dermatitis. Inverse psoriasis presents as well-demarcated erythematous patches and thin plaques with or without white scale. Diagnosis of inverse psoriasis is usually clinical; however, a biopsy can confirm the diagnosis.[38]

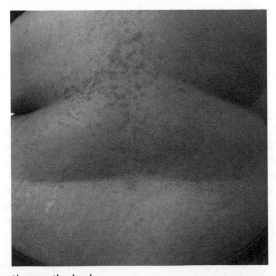

Fig. 8. CARP presenting on the back.

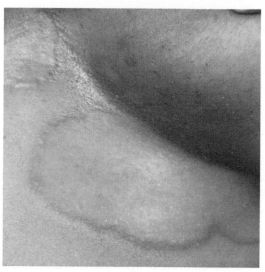

Fig. 9. Inverse psoriasis.

Treatment of psoriasis depends on the degree of disease, areas affected, and presence or absence of joint involvement. In general, mild–moderate plaque psoriasis can usually be managed with topical corticosteroids, vitamin D analogs, or topical calcineurin inhibitors. For inverse psoriasis, first line treatment includes low to mid-potency topical corticosteroids, topical calcineurin inhibitors (tacrolimus or pimecrolimus), or topical vitamin D analogs (calcipotriol) along with emollients. Topical calcineurin inhibitors and vitamin D analogs are the treatment of choice for the inframammary area and nipple because they are less likely to cause skin atrophy as they do not affect collagen synthesis.[38] While systemic and biologic therapies, such as adalimumab and ustekinumab, are commonly used in generalized recalcitrant plaque psoriasis, few studies have been performed for isolated inverse psoriasis.[38,39]

Morphea

Morphea, also known as localized scleroderma, is an inflammatory disease that leads to cutaneous fibrosis and, in certain subtypes, internal involvement. Morphea is more common in women than men and increases in prevalence with increasing age. Cutaneous sclerosis seen in morphea is thought to be due to vascular damage, activated T cells, and altered connective tissue production by fibroblasts. The onset of morphea is likely caused by a triggering event, such as mechanical trauma, injections, or radiation.

The most common variant of morphea, plaque-type, presents as erythematous or violaceous plaques on the trunk. Initially, the lesions can be asymptomatic. The plaques will gradually increase in size and become shiny and sclerotic, often with a violaceous border and atrophic center. As sclerosis progresses, the adnexa is also affected, and the areas become anhidrotic and hairless. Patients may also notice both hypo and hyperpigmentation, and telangiectasias of the affected area.[40]

On the breast, it has been shown that morphea can be triggered by radiation therapy. Postirradiation morphea (PIM) has been described as sudden onset sclerosis of the skin at least 1 month to several years after radiotherapy treatments. Prevalence of PIM is 1 in 3000 cases of postbreast cancer radiation. The sclerosis is typically limited to the irradiated area and the nipple and areola are spared.[41,42] PIM is clinically and histologically indistinguishable from morphea; however, patients will have a history of radiation to the affected area.

Management of morphea, including PIM, includes skin biopsy to confirm diagnosis and treatment manage symptoms and prevent progression of disease. It must be distinguished from lichen sclerosis which initially presents as bluish-white papules and polygonal plaques. Like morphea, these lesions evolve into scar-like plaques with telangiectasias and an atrophic or wrinkled surface. Development of lichen sclerosus has been seen after the treatment of breast cancer with anastrozole and radiation therapy.[43] Li and colleagues also showed an increased prevalence of breast cancer in patients with lichen sclerosus.[44] Initial treatment options include topical corticosteroids for both morphea and lichen sclerosis.[40] Systemic treatment options for severe cases include methotrexate, pentoxifylline, oral corticosteroids, or acitretin.[40,42,45]

Hyperkeratosis of the Nipple and Areola

Hyperkeratosis of the nipple and areola (HNA) is a benign condition characterized by the unilateral or bilateral development of hyperpigmented verrucous papules and plaques involving the nipple and areola. Lesions can affect both men and women but are mostly seen in postpubertal women. A variant of HNA has also been described in pregnancy and during the postpartum period.[46,47] The pathogenesis is unclear; however, because HNA is typically seen postpuberty and similar lesions are seen during pregnancy, the disease may be hormonally driven. Although HNA is typically asymptomatic or mildly pruritic, it will persist without therapy. Treatment options include 6% salicylic acid gel, 2% lactic acid lotion, mild topical corticosteroids, and topical retinoic acids. Cryotherapy, carbon dioxide laser treatment, and surgical removal have also been used in refractory cases.[46,47]

Radiation Dermatitis

Radiation dermatitis (RD) is seen in almost all patients undergoing radiotherapy. The onset of acute RD is typically in the first-fourth weeks of treatment and presentation can be polymorphic and range from mild erythema with hyperpigmentation to moist desquamation, ulceration, and necrosis.[22,48] Management of radiation dermatitis is centered around prevention with sun-protective measures and gentle skin care. Treatment options include the use of hydrocortisone 1% cream or mometasone 0.1% cream. Although topical steroids can be used for symptom control, they have not been shown to prevent the development of acute radiation dermatitis.[49] XonRID, a recently developed water-based gel, may be useful in the prevention of acute dermatitis in the future.[48]

Pemphigus Vulgaris & Paraneoplastic Pemphigus

Pemphigus is a group of autoimmune blistering disorder in which IgG antibodies target proteins in the epidermis. There are 3 major forms of pemphigus including pemphigus foliaceous (PF), pemphigus vulgaris (PV), and paraneoplastic pemphigus (PNP). In PF, patients develop crusted erythematous erosions primarily in a seborrheic distribution on the scalp, face, chest, and back. In PV, flaccid bullae, painful erosions on mucosal surfaces and body can be seen.[50] PNP can present in conjunction with many underlying neoplasms. The most common initial presentation of PNP is severe, recalcitrant hemorrhagic stomatitis. Patients will also present other mucosal and cutaneous involvement similar to PV.[50] PNP has been seen in conjunction with breast adenocarcinoma and is associated with tamoxifen use.[51,52] Diagnosis of diseases in the pemphigus family is performed via clinical examination, H&E skin biopsy, and direct immunofluorescence (DIF). Patients should be referred to a dermatologist for management. Based on the severity of disease, treatment options include topical corticosteroids, oral steroids, and immunosuppressive agents including azathioprine, mycophenolate mofetil, and rituximab (b29). In the cases of PNP, diagnosis and aggressive treatment of the underlying malignancy leads to the improvement of PNP.[51]

Raynaud's Phenomenon

Raynaud's phenomenon (RP) is episodic vasospasm of arteries secondary to various triggers. Risk factors include cold climate, nicotine use, and family history. It can be primary, typically seen in healthy, young females, or secondary, associated with underlying medical problems such as systemic sclerosis.[53,54] RP is typically seen in the fingers and toes but also can involve the branches of the internal and external mammary arteries of the nipple.[53] RP affecting the nipple can present in up to 22% of women of childbearing age and is more common in pregnant and lactating women.[54] It is thought that elevated estrogen levels and emotional stress contribute to the development of RP. RP of the nipple will present as intermittent, sharp, severe nipple pain and discoloration.[54] Diagnosis of RP is clinical and treatment is directed at prevention. Patients should be encouraged to avoid cold climates, optimize stress management, and stop using tobacco. Medical therapies include calcium channel blockers (CCBs), such as nifedipine or amlodipine, both of which are safe to use during breastfeeding. In cases refractory to CCBs, phosphodiesterase type 5 inhibitors, angiotensin receptor blockers, and topical nitroglycerin have been used as well.[55]

Calciphylaxis

Calciphylaxis, also known as calcific uremic arteriolopathy, involves macrocalcifications and occlusion of arterioles, leading to ischemia and necrosis of the affected tissues. It is typically seen in adults with end-stage renal disease or warfarin use in areas of increased adipose tissue, such as the abdomen, buttocks, thighs, and breasts. Presentation can vary to include livedo reticularis, painful subcutaneous induration, ulceration, and necrosis with eschar formation. Livedo reticularis presents as erythematous-violaceous reticulated patches. Lesions are also prone to secondary infection. On the breast, calciphylaxis can lead to peau d'orange changes, mimicking an inflammatory breast cancer.[56,57] Diagnosis can be made with biopsy and through microcalcifications seen on imaging. Patients who present with calciphylaxis on the breast should undergo mammography and sonography. Prognosis is guarded as this condition has a high mortality rate. Treatment of calciphylaxis is multidisciplinary and aimed at symptom management with pain control, wound care, and treatment of contributing conditions. Underlying calcium and phosphate derangements should be managed with hemodialysis or use of calcium and phosphate binders. Sodium thiosulfate and pentoxifylline have been used in the management of calciphylaxis as well.[56–58]

SUMMARY

Based on the number of dermatologic conditions that can present in the breast, it is useful to have a basic working knowledge of such conditions for anyone involved in the care of the breast. Skin biopsy can often be useful in the diagnosis. Referral to dermatology is indicated for many of these conditions.

CRITICAL CARE POINTS/PEARLS AND PITFALLS

- Allergic contact dermatitis can be seen with the use of medical supplies including Dermabond, personal care items, and jewelry
- Psoriasis on the breast presents as nonscaly erythematous plaques in the inframammary fold
- Initial treatment of morphea is topical steroids.
- Any blistering disorders should be biopsied for H&E and direct immunofluorescence to establish the diagnosis as treatment plans can differ.

DISCLOSURE

Dr A.D. Throckmorton has the following disclosures Saunders/Mosby-Elsevier (spouse), Exactech (Spouse), Zimmer (spouse), OsteoCentrics (spouse), Pacira (spouse), Responsive Arthroscopy (spouse), Gilead (self, spouse), Targeted Medical Education (self). Drs S. Pulusani and E. Jones have none.

REFERENCES

1. Requena LRC, Cockerell CJ. Benign Epidermal Tumors and Proliferations. In: Bolognia JL, Schaffer JV, Cerroni L, editors. Dermatology. Philadelphia: Elsevier Limited; 2018. p. 1894–916.
2. Al Ghazal P, Korber A, Klode J, et al. Leser-Trelat sign and breast cancer. Lancet 2013;381(9878):1653.
3. Peters MS, Lehman JS, Comfere NI. Dermatopathology of the female breast. Am J Dermatopathol 2013;35(3):289–304 [quiz 305–7].
4. Fouad TM, Barrera AMG, Reuben JM, et al. Inflammatory breast cancer: a proposed conceptual shift in the UICC-AJCC TNM staging system. Lancet Oncol 2017;18(4):e228–32.
5. NCCN Guidelines for Breast Cancer. Available at: https://www.nccn.org/professionals/physician_gls/pdf/breast.pdf. Accessed January 30, 2022.
6. Dawood S, Merajver SD, Viens P, et al. International expert panel on inflammatory breast cancer: consensus statement for standardized diagnosis and treatment. Ann Oncol 2011;22(3):515–23.
7. Hao X, Billings SD, Wu F, et al. Dermatofibrosarcoma Protuberans: Update on the Diagnosis and Treatment. J Clin Med 2020;9(6). https://doi.org/10.3390/jcm9061752.
8. Wang Y, Wang Y, Chen R, et al. A Rare Malignant Disease, Dermatofibrosarcoma Protuberans of the Breast: A Retrospective Analysis and Review of Literature. Biomed Res Int 2020;2020:8852182.
9. NCCN Guidelines for Dermatofibrosarcoma Protuberans. https://nccn.org/guidelines/guidelines-detail?category=1&id=1430 Accessed January 30, 2022.
10. Gruber P, Zito PM. Skin cancer. Treasure Island, FL: StatPearls; 2022.
11. Goddard L, Mollet T, Blalock T. Resident rounds part III: plaque on left areola of an African-American woman. J Drugs Dermatol 2014;13(6):767.
12. Ferguson MS, Nouraei SA, Davies BJ, et al. Basal cell carcinoma of the nipple-areola complex. Dermatol Surg 2009;35(11):1771–5.
13. Narayanamurthy V, Padmapriya P, Noorasafrin A, et al. Skin cancer detection using non-invasive techniques. RSC Adv 2018;8:28095–130.

14. Dinnes J, Deeks JJ, Chuchu N, et al. Dermoscopy, with and without visual inspection, for diagnosing melanoma in adults. Cochrane Database Syst Rev 2018;12: CD011902.
15. Snashall E, Kiernan T, Harper-Machin A, et al. Primary Melanoma of the Breast Parenchyma: An Oncoplastic Approach. Plast Reconstr Surg Glob Open 2020; 8(12):e3276.
16. Keung EZ, Gershenwald JE. Clinicopathological Features, Staging, and Current Approaches to Treatment in High-Risk Resectable Melanoma. J Natl Cancer Inst 2020;112(9):875–85.
17. Hudson A, Sturgeon A, Peiris A. Tinea Versicolor. JAMA 2018;320(13):1396.
18. Elewski BEHL, Hunt KM, Hay RJ. Fungal Diseases. In: Bolognia JL, Schaffer JV, Cerroni L, editors. Dermatology. Philadelphia: Elsevier Limited; 2018. p. 1329–63.
19. Downing CMN, Sra K, Tyring S. Human Herpesviruses. In: Bolognia JL, Schaffer JV, Cerroni L, editors. Dermatology. Philadelphia: Elsevier Limited; 2018. p. 1400–24.
20. Saunte DML, Jemec GBE. Hidradenitis Suppurativa: Advances in Diagnosis and Treatment. JAMA 2017;318(20):2019–32.
21. Goldburg SR, Strober BE, Payette MJ. Hidradenitis suppurativa: Current and emerging treatments. J Am Acad Dermatol 2020;82(5):1061–82.
22. Waldman RA, Finch J, Grant-Kels JM, et al. Skin diseases of the breast and nipple: Inflammatory and infectious diseases. J Am Acad Dermatol 2019;80(6): 1483–94.
23. Vossen A, van der Zee HH, Prens EP. Hidradenitis Suppurativa: A Systematic Review Integrating Inflammatory Pathways Into a Cohesive Pathogenic Model. Front Immunol 2018;9:2965.
24. Tuffaha SH, Sarhane KA, Mundinger GS, et al. Pyoderma Gangrenosum After Breast Surgery: Diagnostic Pearls and Treatment Recommendations Based on a Systematic Literature Review. Ann Plast Surg 2016;77(2):e39–44.
25. Cabanas Weisz LM, Vicario Elorduy E, Garcia Gutierrez JJ. Pyoderma gangrenosum of the breast: A challenging diagnosis. Breast J 2020;26(11):2188–93.
26. Turcu G, Ioana Nedelcu R, Teodora Nedelcu I, et al. Pyoderma gangrenosum and suppurative hidradenitis association, overlap or spectrum of the same disease? Case report and discussion. Exp Ther Med 2020;20(1):38–41.
27. McAleer M, O'Regan GM, Irvine A. Atopic Dermatitis. In: Bolognia JL, SJ, Cerroni L, editors. Dermatology. Philadelphia: Elsevier Limited; 2018. p. 208–27.
28. Puri A, Sethi A, Puri K, et al. Correlation of nipple eczema in pregnancy with atopic dermatitis in Northern India: a study of 100 cases. An Bras Dermatol 2019;94(5):549–52.
29. Sidbury R, Davis DM, Cohen DE, et al. Guidelines of care for the management of atopic dermatitis: section 3. Management and treatment with phototherapy and systemic agents. J Am Acad Dermatol 2014;71(2):327–49.
30. Ariens LFM, van der Schaft J, Spekhorst LS, et al. Dupilumab shows long-term effectiveness in a large cohort of treatment-refractory atopic dermatitis patients in daily practice: 52-Week results from the Dutch BioDay registry. J Am Acad Dermatol 2021;84(4):1000–9.
31. Nixon RLMC, Marks JG Jr. Allergic Contact Dermatitis. In: Bolognia JL, Schaffer JV, Cerroni L, editors. Dermatology. Philadelphia: Elsevier Limited; 2018. p. 242–61.
32. Kim SK, Won YH, Kim SJ. Nipple eczema: a diagnostic challenge of allergic contact dermatitis. Ann Dermatol 2014;26(3):413–4.

33. Nakagawa S, Uda H, Sarukawa S, et al. Contact Dermatitis Caused by Derma-bond Advanced Use. Plast Reconstr Surg Glob Open 2018;6(9):e1841.
34. Cohen DE. Irritant Contact Dermatitis. In: Bolognia JLSJ, Cerroni L, editors. Dermatology. Philadelphia: Elsevier Limited; 2018. p. 262–73.
35. Reider N, FPOEEIBJ, Schaffer JV, Cerroni L, editors. Dermatology. Elsevier Limited; 2018. p. 228–41.
36. Mufti A, Sachdeva M, Maliyar K, et al. Treatment outcomes in confluent and retic-ulated papillomatosis: A systematic review. J Am Acad Dermatol 2021;84(3): 825–9.
37. van de Kerkhof PCM, NFPIBJ, Schaffer JV, et al, editors. Dermatology. Philadel-phia: Elsevier Limited; 2018. p. 138–60.
38. Micali G, Verzi AE, Giuffrida G, et al. Inverse Psoriasis: From Diagnosis to Current Treatment Options. Clin Cosmet Investig Dermatol 2019;12:953–9.
39. Reynolds KA, Pithadia DJ, Lee EB, et al. Treatments for inverse psoriasis: a sys-tematic review. J Dermatolog Treat 2020;31(8):786–93.
40. Röcken M, GKMaLSIBJ, Schaffer JV, et al, editors. Dermatology. Elsevier Limited; 2018. p. 707–21.
41. Partl R, Regitnig P, Lukasiak K, et al. Incidence of Morphea following Adjuvant Irradiation of the Breast in 2,268 Patients. Breast Care (Basel) 2020;15(3):246–52.
42. Bishnoi A, Kumar S, Handa S, et al. Morphea of the breast: A rare occurrence. Breast J 2019;25(5):1010–1.
43. Vujovic O. Lichen sclerosus in a radiated breast. CMAJ 2010;182(18):E860.
44. Li X, Dooley SW, Patton TJ. Increased prevalence of breast cancer in female pa-tients with lichen sclerosus. J Am Acad Dermatol 2021;84(1):178–80.
45. Friedman O, Barnea Y, Hafner A. Underdiagnosed and disfiguring - Radiation-induced morphea following breast cancer treatment. Breast 2018;39:97–100.
46. Baykal C, Buyukbabani N, Kavak A, et al. Nevoid hyperkeratosis of the nipple and areola: a distinct entity. J Am Acad Dermatol 2002;46(3):414–8.
47. Kar SSP, Yadav N, Bonde P. Pregnancy-associated hyperkeratosis of the nipple/ areola. J Mahatma Gandhi Inst Med Sci 2019;24(2):96.
48. Ingargiola R, De Santis MC, Iacovelli NA, et al. A monocentric, open-label ran-domized standard-of-care controlled study of XONRID(R), a medical device for the prevention and treatment of radiation-induced dermatitis in breast and head and neck cancer patients. Radiat Oncol 2020;15(1):193.
49. Kianinia MRM, Mahdavi H, Hemati S. A Double-Blind Randomized Trial on the Effectiveness of Mometasone 0.1% Cream and Hydrocortisone 1% Cream on the Prevention of Acute Radiation Dermatitis in Breast Cancer Patients following Breast Conserving Surgery. Middle East J Cancer 2021;12(3):406–14.
50. Amagai M. Pemphigus. In: Bolognia JLSJ, Cerroni L, editors. Dermatology. Phil-adelphia: Elsevier Limited; 2018. p. 484–509.
51. Ferguson L, Fearfield L. Paraneoplastic pemphigus foliaceus related to underly-ing breast cancer. Clin Exp Dermatol 2018;43(7):817–8.
52. Kaplan I, Hodak E, Ackerman L, et al. Neoplasms associated with paraneoplastic pemphigus: a review with emphasis on non-hematologic malignancy and oral mucosal manifestations. Oral Oncol 2004;40(6):553–62.
53. Jansen S, Sampene K. Raynaud Phenomenon of the Nipple: An Under-Recognized Condition. Obstet Gynecol 2019;133(5):975–7.
54. Di Como J, Tan S, Weaver M, et al. Nipple pain: Raynaud's beyond fingers and toes. Breast J 2020;26(10):2045–7.
55. Anderson PO. Drug Treatment of Raynaud's Phenomenon of the Nipple. Breast-feed Med 2020;15(11):686–8.

56. Hall DJ, Gentile LF, Duckworth LV, et al. Calciphylaxis of the Breast: A Case Report and Literature Review. Breast J 2016;22(5):568–72.
57. George JT, Green L. Calciphylaxis of the breast, mimicking advanced breast cancer with skin involvement. Radiol Case Rep 2021;16(5):1211–5.
58. Jeong HS, Dominguez AR. Calciphylaxis: Controversies in Pathogenesis, Diagnosis and Treatment. Am J Med Sci 2016;351(2):217–27.

Juvenile Benign Diseases of the Breast

Rona Norelius, MD*

KEYWORDS

- Juvenile • Adolescent • Neonatal • Congenital • Breast

KEY POINTS

- Although most breast disorders in juvenile patients are benign, failure to address or alleviate fears of malignant disease or breast deformity can result in serious detriment to the patient's psychological and sexual development and satisfaction.
- Surgical interventions on the juvenile breast should be avoided if possible. If surgery is warranted, care should be taken to avoid unnecessary damage to the breast bud, as this can result in lifelong disfigurement and malfunction.
- Approach to a juvenile patient with a breast mass may be dictated by the resources available and often differs from the algorithm followed for adult patients.

INTRODUCTION

The presence of mammary glands with the ability to manufacture milk to nourish our offspring separates the mammal from all lower classes of vertebrates. The development of this complex epidermal appendage occurs in distinct phases at different stages of the life cycle. This phased development influences the pathology that can present at different ages of life. Before reaching adulthood, most abnormalities of the breast are benign in nature and can be characterized as congenital disorders, developmental disorders, or acquired disorders. The authors delve further into each of these disorder subtypes after a brief discussion of juvenile breast development.

BREAST DEVELOPMENT

The human breast has 2 main components: the stroma, consisting mainly of adipose tissue, originates from mesodermal elements. The stroma provides a structural housing for the parenchymal components of the breast. The parenchyma originates from ectodermal elements and forms a system of branching ducts leading to secretory

Montana Children's Specialists, Logan Health, 202 Conway Drive, Suite 200, Kalispell, MT 59901, USA
* Corresponding author. Rona Norelius, MD202 Conway DriveKalispell, MT 59901.
E-mail address: rnorelius@logan.org

Surg Clin N Am 102 (2022) 1065–1075
https://doi.org/10.1016/j.suc.2022.07.020
0039-6109/22/© 2022 Elsevier Inc. All rights reserved.

surgical.theclinics.com

acini. Ductal development commences in fetal life and halts, or rather pauses, early in childhood. Hormonal stimulation during puberty triggers further differentiation and development.[1] The incredible cellular plasticity of the human breast allows extensive remodeling into and throughout adulthood and is a factor contributing to the development of disease within the breast.[2]

Early in gestation mammary specific progenitor cells develop into a proliferation of epithelial cells on paired ridges on the thorax to form the mammary crest or milk line. This line extends from the axilla to the inguinal region. In normal development, most of the mammary crest involutes with the exception of the paired, solid epithelial masses in the pectoral region at the fourth intercostal space, which form the primary mammary buds.[3] This embryologic evolution helps to understand many congenital disorders of the human breast such as polymastia and polythelia (**Fig. 1**).

Infant Breast Maturation

The human breast undergoes significant morphological and functional changes from birth to 2 years of age as described by Anbazhagan and colleagues.[4] At birth, both genders usually have palpable breast tissue. The amount of breast tissue present at birth varies greatly from individual to individual. In the first few months of life this tissue responds to decreases in maternal estrogens and increases in endogenous prolactin produced by the developing pituitary gland. These hormonal swings can produce findings in the neonatal breast that may be alarming to some new parents and often require reassurance by the medical provider. Usually, by the end of the second year of life the breast tissue has undergone a process of involution, leaving only small ductal structures in a fibroblastic stroma that remain quiescent until puberty.[5]

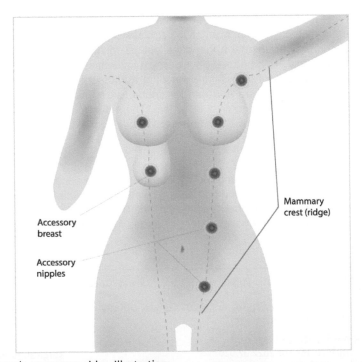

Mammary crest (ridge)

Accessory breast

Accessory nipples

Fig. 1. Female mammary ridge illustration.

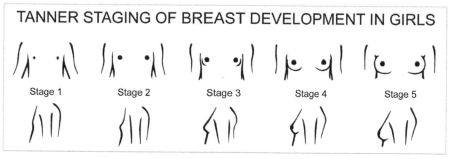

Fig. 2. Tanner stages.

Puberty/Thelarche

Breast development begins between the ages of 8 and 13 years and is often the first sign of puberty in women. Recent reports show that thelarche (or breast budding) is observed at an earlier age than previously documented.[6] The reasons for this are most likely multifactorial and not universally agreed upon at this time. A true diagnosis of precocious puberty requires a complex and multifaceted evaluation, but the onset of secondary breast development prior to age 8 years should alert the medical provider to a possible abnormality and prompt further investigation. Similarly, the lack of thelarche by age 13 years should also prompt further investigation and may signal delayed puberty. Breast abnormalities can occur at any stage in life. Therefore, a breast examination should be considered part of a complete physical examination for all patients, regardless of age.

Tanner Stages

In 1969 Tanner first described the patterns of pubertal changes in girls, thus creating the commonly adopted Tanner staging system used to characterize and define the progression of puberty.[7] When evaluating a juvenile breast disorder it is important to note the Tanner stage, as it is recommended to wait until breast development is complete (Tanner stage V) when intervening upon or treating some benign disorders. Unnecessary intervention, surgical or medical, during early breast development may negatively affect the long-term development or function of the breast with significant cosmetic abnormality or difficulties with lactation. Because the parenchymal components undergo significant growth and maturation during hormonal surges (most notably puberty and pregnancy) a small defect in an undeveloped breast may translate to a large deformity in a mature breast (**Fig. 2**).

CONGENITAL DISORDERS
Malformations of the Breast

Amastia is congenital abscess of the breast (**Box 1**). It is rare and secondary to complete obliteration of the mammary line and may be unilateral or bilateral. At birth there

---

Box 1
Congenital disorders of the breast

- Malformations
  - Amastia
  - Polymastia
  - Athelia
  - Polythelia

- Nipple discharge in the newborn
  - Milky
  - Bloody

- Masses in the neonatal breast
  - Hypertrophy
  - Mastitis/abscess
  - Cyst
  - Hypertrophic lymph node
  - Hemangiomas and lymphangiomas

---

is noted absence of breast tissue and the nipple-areola complex. At puberty, there is lack of breast development but other secondary sexual characteristics will develop normally, and fertility is preserved.[8] Amastia is often associated with other congenital malformations and syndromes. Ninety percent of patients with unilateral amastia also have absence of the pectoralis major muscle (Poland syndrome)[9] (**Table 1**).

Polymastia is a congenital malformation characterized by the development of more than 2 breasts. It occurs in 1% of the population.[6] Polymastia is subdivided into 2 types of malformations: supernumerary breast and aberrant or accessory mammary tissue that forms outside of the mammary line.[9] Complete supernumerary breasts contain all the components of normal breast with well-formed ductal system and nipple areola complex. This finding is extremely rare.[9] More commonly, supernumerary breasts develop ductal systems that lack a nipple areola complex. The most frequent locations are the axilla or vulvo-inguinal region.[9] When a supernumerary breast develops it may evade detection well into adulthood. When situated in a position above the normal breast a supernumerary breast can lactate. All supernumerary breast tissues are subject to the same cyclic changes of development and hormonal influence as normal breasts and, thus, is at risk for all pathologic changes of a normal breast including carcinoma.[10] Some investigators advocate excision of supernumerary and accessory breast tissue to avoid painful swelling in the region with pregnancy and other hormonal swings.

Table 1
Amastia

Amastia	Associated Anomalies
Unilateral	*Poland syndrome:* absence of pectoralis muscle and rib deformities
Bialteral	*Skeletal:* absence of ulna, lobster claw, absence of fingers, syndactyly, clinodactyly, cubitus valgus *Facial:* cleft palate, hypertelorism, macrostomia, low-set ears, hearing defect, multiple whorls *Renal:* ureteral triplication, malrotated kidneys, chronic renal disease *Genital:* hypoplasia of labia majora, vaginal agenesis

Athelia is congenital absence of the nipple. It is a very rare disorder and occurs more frequently when accessory breast tissue develops along the mammary line. There are, however, case reports of athelia in primary breast development.[11] The nipple complex does not develop until the eighth month of gestation, making it difficult to identify in the premature infant; therefore, invasive procedures on premature infants such as central line placement or chest tube placement may permanently impede the development of a normal nipple.

Polythelia is congenital presence of more than 2 nipples. These supernumerary nipples usually develop along the milk line. Resection of accessory nipples can be performed for cosmetic reasons. There is an association between the presence of supernumerary nipples and anomalies of the kidney and urinary tract (including functional disorders, malformations and congenital disease); therefore, if polythelia is present it should prompt a workup with a renal ultrasound.[12]

Nipple Discharge in the Newborn

Up to 5% of newborns may experience a transient secretion of milky liquid from their nipples; this may be unilateral or bilateral and results from the falling maternal estrogens, which, in turn, stimulates the neonatal pituitary gland to produce prolactin.[4,5] This milk is colloquially termed "witch's milk." The term comes from ancient folklore that fluid leaking from a newborn's nipple was a source of nourishment for witches' familiar spirits. It can be seen in infants of either gender, is associated with larger than average breast buds, and can persist until 2 months of age. It is more common in infants who are breast fed and rarely seen in premature infants. It is a benign finding that should be treated only with reassurance to the caregivers and observation on the part of the medical provider.[13]

Bloody nipple discharge in the infant occurs much less frequently and is usually the result of mammary duct ectasia. This bloody discharge usually presents later than the milky discharge seen in neonates. Patients may be a few months old when this is first noted, and there may or may not be a palpable lesion within the breast tissue. Historically, when these lesions have been biopsied, the histology shows dilated ducts surrounded by fibrosis and inflammation.[14] Biopsy for bloody nipple discharge in an infant is no longer routinely recommended. Mammary duct ectasia is a benign and self-limiting disorder that may persist for up to 9 months.[15] Surgical resection within that window is not advised, as removal of part of the breast bud will almost certainly result in permanent disfigurement and possible functional issues.

Masses in the Neonatal Breast

There are many breast masses that present in neonatal life, including hypertrophic breast tissue, mastitis and breast abscesses, cysts, and hypertrophied lymph nodes. All are benign and usually related to hormonal fluctuations and breast tissue remodeling as previously discussed.

Breast hypertrophy can appear as a distinct mass, can be either unilateral or bilateral, and occurs in both male and female neonates. It usually self-resolves within a few weeks in male neonates and within several months in female neonates. Stimulating the breast tissue with massage or attempts to express liquid from the nipple may encourage the hypertrophic tissue to persist or induce infection.

Although rare, neonates can develop infections in the breast tissue. Mastitis is most often seen in the first 2 weeks of life and more often in female than male neonates.[16] In a small review of patient presenting in the first 3 months of life with mastitis, those treated with oral antibiotics all went on to abscess formation[17]; thus, it is recommended that for infants presenting with mastitis treatment is initiated with parenteral antibiotics that cover methicillin-resistant *Staphylococcus aureus*. If an abscess is noted on examination or ultrasound, it may be beneficial to aspirate the purulent fluid and avoid incision and drainage procedures that may permanently damage the breast bud. Occasionally, soft tissue infections in the breast can lead to complex or systemic infections such as necrotizing fasciitis, shock, or CNS involvement. Severe disease such as this arises in less than 2% of infants presenting with mastitis.[18] If the infant is febrile or ill-appearing, a full workup should be undertaken, looking for deeper or additional sites of infection.

Other masses that can present in the neonatal breast tissue include cysts or hypertrophic lymph nodes. Ultrasound characteristics can usually differentiate these 2 entities and can be used to track growth or changes if needed at intervals of 6 to 12 weeks. Surgical intervention is very rarely indicated and most neonatal breast cysts will self-resolve.

Hemangiomas and lymphangiomas may also be mistaken for enlarging breasts or breast masses in young children. If in doubt, an ultrasound study with Doppler or MRI can provide a diagnosis. Surgical excision is not indicated. Rapid growth may warrant evaluation and treatment (usually with minimally invasive endovascular techniques) in a center with expertise in pediatric lymphovascular malformations.

DEVELOPMENTAL DISORDERS
Premature or Delayed Thelarche

Thelarche, or breast development, typically begins between the ages of 8 and 13 years with an average age of onset of 10.3 years **Box 2**.[19] As previously discussed, normal breast tissue undergoes initial development with regression in the first two years of life. However, breast development between the ages of 2 and 8 is considered abnormal and warrants investigation for premature or precocious puberty with evaluation of clinical, hormonal, and radiographic parameters. If precocious puberty is not evident, an ultrasound of the breast tissue is recommended to evaluate for an underlying mass or growth within the breast causing the appearance of breast development. On the other hand, if there is no evidence of breast development by age 13 years, the patient should be referred for a workup for delayed puberty.[20]

Atrophy

Significant and rapid weight loss leading to loss of adipose tissue is the most common cause of breast atrophy in the juvenile patient; this may be secondary to anorexia

---

Box 2
Developmental disorders of the breast

- Premature thelarche
- Delayed thelarche
- Breast atrophy
- Hypomastia/micromastia
- Juvenile breast hypertrophy
- Breast shape variation
  - Asymmetry
  - Tuberous breasts
- Male gynecomastia

nervosa or other chronic condition leading to malnutrition. Other causes of breast atrophy include scleroderma and early ovarian failure, resulting in a premature decrease in circulating estrogen levels.[21] In addition, localized atrophy of breast tissue may occur secondary to blunt force trauma. Traumatic injury to the breast tissue may induce necrosis of the soft tissue, leading to focal atrophy.

Hypomastia/Micromastia

Underdevelopment or failure of development of normal breasts despite the presence of mammary gland tissue is termed hypomastia or micromastia. The cause of this disorder is not well understood. It may be unilateral or bilateral or syndromic or nonsyndromic. There are reports of hypomastia following thoracic radiation, interventions that damage the breast bud early in childhood such as placement of chest tubes in undeveloped chests, and burns to the anterior chest wall.[22] The mammary tissue in cases of breast hypoplasia consists of fibrous stroma and ductal structures without acinar differentiation.[23] Referral to a reconstructive breast surgeon is usually indicated, as treatment involves breast augmentation. Optimal timing of surgical intervention is debated. Many surgeons advocate waiting until breast development is complete (age 18 years or tanner stage IV) to initiate surgical intervention but there can be psychosocial detriments to proceeding through adolescence without normal breast development. Some investigators also argue for earlier intervention with acknowledgment that revisional surgery may be necessary as the child ages and grows.[24]

Juvenile Breast Hypertrophy

Massive and rapid development of one or both breasts despite normal levels of circulating estrogens is termed juvenile, virginal, or idiopathic breast hypertrophy.[21] It is a rare disorder that usually presents as an alarmingly rapid growth of excessive breast tissue over a 6-month period (often 1–2 years before menarche) followed by a period of slower and more consistent growth.[25,26] There are many theories about the cause of this rapid and massive development of breast tissue. A few common theories include an abnormal ratio of estrogens to progesterone or abnormal sensitivity to estrogen in the breast tissue.[21,27] There is no medically approved treatment in children; therefore; surgical breast reduction is usually indicated, as the breast tissue can reach a weight of up to 20 kg and can lead to significant psychosocial and physical discomfort. Unfortunately, breast reduction is associated with high rates of recurrence.[27]

Breast Shape Variation

Each breast arises from an individual breast bud; therefore, there is almost always some asymmetry in development, which is usually mild and remains unnoticed. Significant asymmetry may cause significant deformity and may require surgical correction with augmentation of the smaller breast or reduction of the larger breast. This cosmetic procedure should generally be delayed until full development is reached to optimize outcomes. Breast tissue asymmetry should also be differentiated from pseudo-asymmetry in which an illusion of inequality is due to scoliosis or a chest wall deformity.[6] Treatment of pseudo-asymmetry may also require reshaping of the chest wall to achieve optimal results.

There is significant variation is breast shape and size, which is influenced by factors such as race and body construction. There are many descriptors for different breast shapes such as discoidal, hemispheric, pear-shaped, conical, and tuberous.[8] The tuberous breast (also termed herniated areolar complex, tubular breast, narrow-based breast, snoopy deformity, and lower-pole hypoplastic breast) is one of the most challenging developmental variations.[28] There is wide variation in the appearance, classification, and treatment recommendations and options for women with a tuberous breast deformity; therefore, evaluation and management by a plastic surgeon with expertise in tuberous breast reconstruction is recommended.

MALE GYNECOMASTIA is addressed in a separate article in this publication.

Acquired disorders

Infections. Breast infections tend to occur in 2 distinct age groups in children: first in the neonatal period, as previously discussed, and again around the time of adolescence (**Box 3**).[29] Many of the causes in the 2 patient populations are similar, as these are periods of development with great hormonal variation. In the pubescent population self-inflicted trauma, such as nipple piercings, can lead to mastitis or breast abscess. The pathogens are quite similar between the 2 groups, with the majority of infections caused by S aureus and a smaller number attributable to gram-negative bacilli, group A Streptococcus, and enterococcus.[29] In the neonate, it is recommended to initiate treatment with parenteral antibiotics because there is a risk of systemic spread of infection in the weak neonatal immune system. In an adolescent presenting with mastitis it is acceptable to begin treatment with oral antibiotics and monitor for response. Antibiotic choice should be governed by culture results, if available. If no culture results are available, the regimen should cover gram-positive cocci and gram-negative organisms according to local susceptibility patterns. In the adolescent population most providers are quicker to perform incision and drainage procedures if a large abscess is present. It is still recommended to minimize damage to the breast bud and ductal structures as much as possible in the maturing breast by making a small periareolar incision and probing as little as possible.

Masses in the adolescent breast. The adolescent breast undergoes significant growth and change during puberty, and it is not uncommon to palpate abnormal growths within the developing breast tissue; this can be worrisome for the patient and their family, so it is important to remember and counsel families that most masses in the adolescent breast are benign. In fact, only 0.02% to 0.5% of masses in women under the age of 20 years are malignant.[6,30]

Fibrocystic changes. Cyclic changes in breast size during menstruation can result in mastodynia, and tenderness in the premenstrual period is common and most consistent with fibrocystic changes in the adolescent breast.[31] Physical examination may reveal diffuse, firm, and mobile nodules spread throughout the breast tissue. Ultrasound examination may be obtained to aid with diagnosis and can be a useful adjunct; however, ultrasound has shown to be normal in up to 59% of adolescents with complaints of palpable breast abnormality and pain.[32] Treatment is supportive and consists of heat, analgesics, supportive clothing, and hormone regulation with oral contraceptives. Symptoms will usually resolve as puberty progresses.

Box 3
Acquired disorders of the adolescent breast

- Infections
- Masses
  - Fibrocystic changes
  - Solid masses
- Trauma/hematoma
- Nipple discharge

Solid breast masses in the juvenile patient. The prevalence of breast masses in teenage girls is 3.2% (**Fig. 3**).[33] Although the differential diagnosis for pediatric breast masses is similar to those in adults, the vast majority of breast masses in pediatric patients are benign. Ninety-five percent of surgically removed pediatric breast masses are benign fibroadenomas.[30] Fibroadenomas usually present as a 2- to 3-cm mobile and rubbery round or ovoid mass in the upper, outer quadrant of the breast; however, fibroadenomas can present in any quadrant and may grow quite large. In addition, multiple fibroadenomas occur in 10% to 25% of cases.[34] A suggested workup algorithm is outlined in the accompanying chart (Approach to the Juvenile Breast Mass). Solid breast masses less than 4 cm in diameter that are otherwise asymptomatic can usually be observed for at least 1 menstrual cycle/month. If the mass is persistent, ultrasound and physical examination should be performed at 6- to 12-month intervals. Masses that greater than 4 cm, or have concerning findings on ultrasound, or are symptomatic should be biopsied or excised.

Fine-needle aspiration (FNA) is not recommended in the adolescent population, as FNA samples cannot reliably distinguish between phyllodes tumor and fibroadenoma, and inaccurate diagnosis may be made based on a sampling error. Therefore, if tissue diagnosis is desired or indicated, core needle biopsy or excisional biopsy is recommended. Although core needle biopsy is used routinely in the adult population, special consideration needs to be given when considering core needle biopsy in the juvenile patient. Most invasive procedures in pediatric patients are performed under sedation or general anesthesia for the safety of the patient and the practitioner. Most breast centers that offer expertise in the core needle biopsy technique are not equipped to meet the psychosocial needs of many adolescents requiring invasive procedures. Therefore, it is a common and acceptable practice among pediatric surgeons to offer open excisional under general anesthesia of masses that meet criteria for histologic evaluation or when patients and families feel strongly about obtaining a tissue diagnosis for psychological well-being.

When excising a solid mass in a juvenile patient care must be taken to avoid collateral damage to the still developing breast. Many lesions can effectively be excised through a circumareolar incision. If the lesion is far away from the areola an inframammary, curvilinear or semilunar incision directly over the mass may be used.

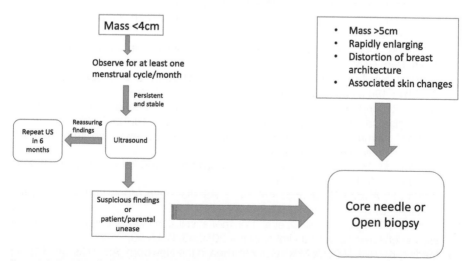

Fig. 3. Approach to the juvenile breast mass.

Trauma. Trauma to the juvenile breast is managed similarly to that in the adult patient.[35] Hematoma development occurs early in the course following blunt breast trauma and can lead to fat necrosis with cosmetic deformity. Greater than 90% of blunt injuries to breast tissue can be managed expectantly, with the minority requiring intervention via either angiographic arterial embolization or open control of bleeding vessels.[36] Most nonexpanding hematomas will self-resolve with time and do not require open evacuation.

NIPPLE DISCHARGE is addressed in a separate article in this publication.

CLINICS CARE POINTS

- Neonatal mastitis should first be treated with parenteral antibiotics with coverage for *S aureus*.
- The primary imaging modality for juvenile breast masses is ultrasound.
- Greater than 95% of solid breast masses in pediatric patients are benign and can be observed without surgical intervention.
- Surgical interventions that disrupt the breast bud can lead to life-long disfigurement.

DISCLOSURE

The author has nothing to disclose.

REFERENCES

1. Sternlicht MD. Key stages in mammary gland development: the cues that regulate ductal branching morphogenesis. Breast Cancer Res 2006;8(1):201.
2. Javed A, Lteif A. Development of the human breast. Semin Plast Surg 2013; 27(1):5–12.
3. Seltzer V. The Breast: embryology, development, and antomy. Clin Obstet Gynecol 1994;37(4):879–80.
4. Anbazhagan R, Bartek J, Monaghan P, et al. Growth and development of the human infant breast. Am J Anat 1991;192(4):407–17.
5. Mckiernan JF, Hull D. Breast development in the newborn. Arch Dis Child 1981; 56(7):525–9.
6. Greydanus DE, Matytsina L, Gains M. Breast disorders in children and adolescents. Prim Care 2006;33:455.
7. Marshall WA, Tanner JM. Variations in pattern of pubertal changes in girls. Arch Dis Child 1969;44(235):291–303.
8. Merlob P. Congenital malformations and developmental changes of the breast: a neonatological view. J Pediatr Endocrinol Metab 2003;16(4):471–85.
9. Trier WC. Complete breast absence: case report and review of the literature. Plast Reconstr Surg 1965;36:431–9.
10. Goedert JJ, McKeen EA, Fraumeni JF. Polymastia and renal adenocarcinoma. Ann Intern Med 1981;95:182–4.
11. Ishida LH, Alves HR, Munhoz AM, et al. Athelia: case report and review of the literature. Br J Plast Surg 2005;58(6):833–7.
12. Ferrara P, Giorgio V, Vitelli O, et al. Polythelia: still a marker of urinary tract anomalies in children? Scand J Urol Nephrol 2009;43(1):47–50.
13. Madlon-Kay DJ. 'Witch's Milk': Galactorrhea in the Newborn. Am J Dis Child 1986; 140(3):252–3.

14. Imamoglu M, Cay A, Reis A, et al. Bloody nipple discharge in children: possible etiologies and selection of appropriate therapy. Pediatr Surg Int 2006;22(2):158–63.
15. Ujiie H, Akiyama M, Osawa R, et al. Bloody Nipple Discharge in an infant. Arch Dermatol 2009;145(9):1068–9.
16. Efrat M, Mogilner JG, Lujtman M, et al. Neonatal mastitis – diagnosis and treatment. Isr J Med Sci 1995;31:558–60.
17. Stricker T, Navratil F, Sennhauser FH. Mastitis in early infancy. Acta Paediatr 2005; 94(2):166–9.
18. Kaplan RL, Cruz AT, Michelson KA, et al. Neonatal mastitis and concurrent serious bacterial infection. Pediatrics 2021;148(1). e2021051322.
19. Biro FM, Greenspan LC, Galvez MP, et al. Onset of breast development in a longitudinal cohort. Pediatrics 2013;132(6):1019–27.
20. Kaplowitz P, Bloch C. Section on Endocrinology, American Academy of Pediatrics. Evaluation and referral of children with signs of early puberty. Pediatrics 2016;137(1):1–6.
21. Mareti E, Vatopoulou A, Spyropoulou GA, et al. Breast disorders in adolescence: a review of the literature. Breast Care (Basel) 2021;16(2):149–55.
22. Latham K, Fernandez S, Iteld L, et al. Pediatric breast deformity. J Craniofac Surg 2006;17(3):454–67.
23. Rosen PP. Rosen's breast pathology. 2nd ed. Philadelphia (PA): Lippincott Williams &Wilkins; 2001. p. 23–9.
24. Oakes MB, Quint EH, Smith YR, et al. Early, staged reconstruction in young women with severe breast asymmetry. J Pediatr Adolesc Gynecol 2009;22(4):223–8.
25. Uribe Barreto A. Juvenile mammary hypertrophy. Plast Reconstr Surg 1991;87(3): 583–4.
26. Kupfer D, Dingman D, Broadbent R. Juvenile breast hypertrophy: report of a familial pattern and review of the literature. Plast Reconstr Surg 1992;90(2):303–9.
27. Wolfswinkel EM, Lemaine V, Weathers WM, et al. Hyperplastic breast anomalies in the female adolescent breast. Semin Plast Surg 2015;135(1):73–86.
28. Winocour S, Lemaine V. Hypoplastic breast anomalies in the female adolescent breast. Semin Plast Surg 2013;27(1):42–8.
29. Faden H. Mastitis in children from birth to 17 years. Pediatr Infect Dis J 2005; 24(12):1113.
30. Simmons PS, Jayasinghe YL, Wold LE, et al. Breast carcinoma in young women. Obstet Gynecol 2011;118(3):529–36.
31. Neinstein LS. Review of breast masses in adolescents. Adolesc Pediatr Gynecol 1994;7(3):119–29.
32. Foxcroft LM, Evans EB, Hirst C, et al. Presentation and diagnosis of adolescent breast disease. Breast 2001;10(5):399–404.
33. Neinstein LS, Atkingson J, Diament M. Prevalence and longitudinal study of breast masses in adolescents. J Adolesc Health 1993;14(4):277–81.
34. Diehl T, Kaplan DW. Breast masses in adolescent females. J Adolesc Health Care 1985;695:353–7.
35. Warren R, Degnim AC. Uncommon benign breast abnormalities in adolescents. Semin Plast Surg 2013;27(1):26–8. https://doi.org/10.1055/s-0033-1343993.
36. Sander C, Cipolla J, Stehly C, Hoey B. Blunt breast trauma: is there a standard of care? Am Surg 2011;77(8):1066–9.

Management of Nipple Discharge

Rick D. Vavolizza, MD[1], Lynn T. Dengel, MD, MSc*

KEYWORDS

- Physiologic versus pathologic • Bloody • Nipple discharge

KEY POINTS

- Nipple discharge is the third most common breast-related complaint but is rarely the presenting symptom of breast cancer.
- Nipple discharge is categorized as lactational, physiologic, or pathologic.
- Pathologic nipple discharge is typically unilateral, spontaneous, from a single duct, and can range from bloody to serous.
- Patients with pathologic discharge should undergo age-appropriate imaging workup, most often including mammogram and ultrasound. If initial imaging is negative, additional imaging including MRI, galactogram, and ductoscopy should be considered. Cytologic evaluation of the discharge is not useful.
- All women and men with pathologic nipple discharge should be referred to a breast surgeon for evaluation, treatment, and follow-up.

INTRODUCTION

Nipple discharge is the third most common breast-related complaint, after breast pain and breast mass,[1] with a reported prevalence of 5% to 7%.[1–4] Although nipple discharge frequently causes concern among patients, it is rarely the presenting symptom of breast cancer. Up to 80% of women will report at least one episode of nipple discharge during reproductive years.[5,6] As such, the primary goals of diagnostic workup and management are to distinguish patients with benign, physiologic nipple discharge from those with pathologic nipple discharge, and to treat the later according to the underlying pathologic condition.

The objectives of this review will address the (1) types and causes of nipple discharge, (2) approach to history taking and physical examination, (3) diagnostic workup, and (4) treatment options.

University of Virginia Department of Surgery Breast and Melanoma Surgery Division, P.O. Box 80709, Charlottesville, VA 22908
[1] Present address: 852 West Main Street, Charlottesville, VA 22903.
* Corresponding author. University of Virginia Department of Surgery Breast and Melanoma Surgery Division, P.O. Box 80709, Charlottesville, VA 22908
E-mail address: LTD5B@virginia.edu

Surg Clin N Am 102 (2022) 1077–1087
https://doi.org/10.1016/j.suc.2022.06.006
0039-6109/22/© 2022 Elsevier Inc. All rights reserved.

surgical.theclinics.com

Table 1 Medications that can cause galactorrhea	
Medication Class	**Medication Name**
Antipsychotics (first generation)	Haloperidol Fluphenazine Chlorpromazine
Antipsychotics (second generation)	Risperidone Paliperidone Asenapine
Antidepressants	Clomipramine Amitriptyline
Antiemetics	Metoclopramide Prochlorperazine
Antihypertensives	Methyldopa Verapamil

TYPES AND CAUSES OF NIPPLE DISCHARGE

Nipple discharge is categorized as lactational, physiologic, or pathologic.

Lactational is benign nipple secretion that typically occurs postpartum. During pregnancy and in the postpartum period, a multitude of hormonal changes[7,8] stimulate mammary gland development and milk production. Lactation consultants and physicians alike have reported that milk secretion can last from 6 months to several years after delivery or after cessation of breastfeeding.[9] Some ejection or leakage of colostrum can occur starting in the second trimester (typically around week 20 of gestation); however, the quantity and frequency of this is limited due to high circulating estrogen and progesterone levels that inhibit milk production during pregnancy.[10,11]

Galactorrhea is a benign, physiologic nipple discharge in patients who are not peripartum and not breastfeeding. Galactorrhea most commonly presents as bilateral milky nipple discharge arising from multiple ducts. However, it can also be unilateral and range in color, from yellow (straw-colored), green/brown, to gray but not sanguineous. Galactorrhea is typically caused by hyperprolactinemia due to medications (Table 1)[12–14] but may also be a presenting symptom of pituitary tumors, and endocrine disorders such as hypothyroidism.

Pathologic nipple discharge is typically unilateral (from one breast), arising from a single duct, spontaneous, and persistent. It is commonly serous (clear or straw-colored yellow), bloody, or serosanguineous in color. The most common causes include benign intraductal papilloma (52%–57%)[15–17] and mammary duct ectasia (14%–33%).[15] Breast cancer may also present as bloody nipple discharge but is a less frequent cause (5%–15%).[3,18,19]

Discharge associated with an intraductal papilloma is typically bloody. The vast majority of papillomas are located within 2 cm from the nipple–areola complex.[16]

Mammary duct ectasia presents as green/black, gray, or even white discharge that is associated with pain and tenderness at the nipple and areola.[20] Purulent nipple discharge can also be seen with nonlactational mastitis with or without an abscess.

When an underlying breast cancer is present in a patient with nipple discharge, the discharge is most often bloody. The risk of breast cancer increases with age among those presenting with nipple discharge. Among women with bloody nipple discharge without a palpable mass, breast cancer was present in 3% of patients aged younger than 40 years, 10% of patients aged 40 to 60 years, and 32% of those aged older than 60 years.[21] Male patients with pathologic nipple discharge have a higher incidence of breast cancer than women, ranging from 23% to 57%. In both women and men, the rate of malignancy increases when a clinically palpable or radiologically evident lesion accompanies the nipple discharge.[22–26]

HISTORY AND PHYSICAL EXAMINATION

A clinical history and physical examination should be performed on all patients presenting with nonlactational nipple discharge to differentiate physiologic from pathologic nipple discharge. Key elements of the clinical history include the nipple discharge color (bloody vs nonbloody), unilateral versus bilateral, spontaneous versus nonspontaneous/provoked by manipulation of the breast, single duct versus multiple ducts, and the frequency of the discharge.

Physical examination focuses on the bilateral breast examination, which includes examining the axillary and supraclavicular lymph nodes. Key elements to the breast examination begin with noting symmetry and contours of the breast, masses, skin changes (ie, skin retraction, dimpling, edema, or erythema), nipple retraction, and crusting or ulceration of the nipple–areola complex. Although examining the skin of the breast, it is important to note any lesions at the nipple–areolar complex that may be mimicking nipple discharge such as Paget disease of the breast. As part of the examination, the breast is compressed to determine if the nipple discharge is reproducible, and, if so, the nature of the discharge including color and ductal distribution. To do so, pressure can be applied in a clockwise fashion around the areola[27] working from the periphery of the areola and moving toward the nipple.

DIAGNOSTIC WORKUP

Patients with milky nipple discharge who are lactating should be reassured and informed no further evaluation is needed unless the discharge persists past 6 months after delivery or after cessation of breastfeeding. Up to 20% of pregnant and lactating women may experience bloody nipple discharge (pink tinged to red in color) secondary to the hypervascularity of the developing breast. Diagnostic workup should be pursued if pathologic nipple discharge persists for more than 7 days because most cases are benign and do not require surgical treatment.[28–30]

Patients with physiologic nipple discharge (galactorrhea) should be ensured they are up-to-date on age appropriate routine screening mammograms and then worked up for hyperprolactinemia. Several common medications are known to cause galactorrhea (see Table 1), most commonly antipsychotics and metoclopramide. Laboratory tests should include a pregnancy test in women, prolactin level, and thyroid stimulating hormone (TSH) level with reflexive T3/T4.

All patients with pathologic nipple discharge require age-appropriate breast imaging to evaluate for an underlying lesion. The choice between mammogram or ultrasound or both is dependent on the age and sex of the patient (Fig. 1).[5] Women aged 40 years and older should undergo both diagnostic mammogram and focused breast ultrasound.[5,31,32] Women who have had a recent mammogram in the last 6 months or are currently pregnant can undergo a focused breast ultrasound alone. Women aged 30 to 39 years should undergo a diagnostic mammogram first, followed by a focused breast ultrasound if necessary for further delineation of the retroareolar tissue.[5] Women aged less than 30 years should undergo a focused breast ultrasound first, followed by a diagnostic mammogram if the ultrasound suggests a suspicious finding or if the patient has an increased risk of hereditary breast cancer.[5] Finally,

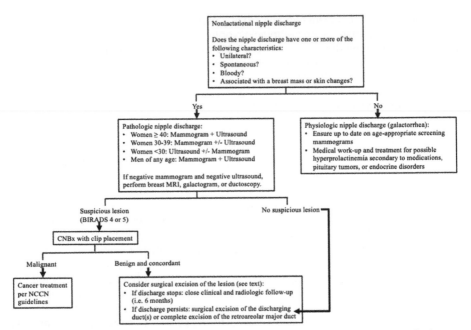

Fig. 1. Diagnostic algorithm for nonlactational nipple discharge. CNBx, core needle biopsy; NCCN, National Comprehensive Cancer Network.

men of any age should undergo both diagnostic mammogram and focused breast ultrasound given the rarity of cases and the higher incidence of underlying breast cancer when men present with pathologic nipple discharge.[32] It is important to note that cytology of pathologic nipple discharge is not recommended because it does not change management[17,33] because abnormal findings do not help with localizing an underlying lesion in the breast. Furthermore, it is technically challenging to differentiate benign, apoptotic cells from atypical cells. A retrospective study of 618 consecutive patients with pathologic nipple discharge found the sensitivity and specificity of nipple discharge cytology to be 17% and 66%, respectively.[17] This study further examined the unique sensitivity and unique specificity of nipple discharge cytology. Unique sensitivity was defined as the proportion of malignancies that were identified exclusively by cytology. Unique specificity was defined as the proportion of benign breast lesions that were designated malignant by examination, mammography and ultrasound but benign by cytology. Only 1 malignant lesion was designated positive exclusively by nipple discharge cytology (unique sensitivity [95% CI], 2.8% [0.0%–8.4%]), and 3 lesions were correctly designated as negative by nipple discharge cytology (unique specificity [95% CI], 1.6% [0.0%–3.7%]).[17] Given the unreliability and little complementary diagnostic value, cytology is not recommended as part of the diagnostic workup for pathologic nipple discharge.

In general, mammography is the imaging modality of choice for identifying suspicious breast lesions. However, mammography can fail to show lesions that lack calcifications, are small in size, are retroareolar, or are completely intraductal.[31,34] Among patients with pathologic nipple discharge, ultrasound can identify 63% to 69% of lesions not seen on mammogram.[25,35] In a study of 106 patients with pathologic nipple discharge, the risk of breast cancer was 3% with a negative mammogram compared with 0% when both mammogram and subareolar ultrasound were negative.[31]

Ultrasound is a valuable imaging modality to diagnose ductal disease by visualizing dilated ducts, wall thickening, intraductal masses, and increased vascularity (**Fig. 2**). Ultrasound can be used to then guide core needle biopsy (CNBx) of palpable lesions or intraductal lesions lacking calcifications. An ultrasound-guided CNBx is a technically easier procedure and provides greater patient comfort compared with that of a stereotactic CNBx.

Patients with pathologic nipple discharge who have a negative mammogram and negative ultrasound should undergo breast MRI, galactogram, or ductoscopy.

Contrast-enhanced MRI is preferred over galactogram and ductoscopy by many health-care providers. MRI has a sensitivity between 93% and 100% for invasive breast cancer and benign papillomas,[36] and specificity between 37%[5] and 85%.[36] The sensitivity and specificity of MRI for ductal carcinoma in situ is 92% to 98%[37] and 76%,[38] respectively. It provides visualization of dilated ducts and nodules within them while providing excellent detail of enhancing lesions.[39] MRI has a higher diagnostic accuracy compared with a galactogram for the detection of breast cancer among patients with pathologic nipple discharge.[40] The sensitivity and specificity of a galactogram is 76% and 11%, respectively,[41] and the absence of a lesion on galactogram does not rule out an underlying malignancy.[41,42] MRI is able to detect lesions attributable to the nipple discharge that are more distant from the nipple. Equally important, galactogram and ductoscopy are less widely available than MRI and can only be performed if the nipple discharge can be reproduced on physical examination, and the target duct diameter is large enough to cannulate. During a galactogram, the opening of the discharging duct is cannulated and injected with a small amount of contrast material. A mammogram is subsequently taken in order to visualize a filling defect or complete obstruction of the duct, if present (**Fig. 3**).[43] If a lesion is identified, then tomosynthesis-guided biopsy is performed on the lesion.

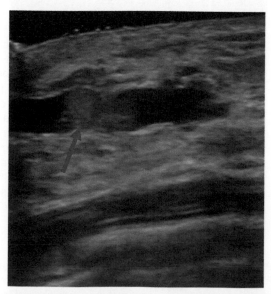

Fig. 2. Breast intraductal papilloma image. Breast ultrasound illustrating a dilated duct and soft tissue echoes within the duct suggestive of an intraluminal lesion (*arrow*). These findings are consistent with an intraductal papilloma. (Original figure courtesy of Jonathan Nguyen, MD.)

Following radiologic localization of a suspicious breast lesion, image-guided CNBx with postbiopsy clip placement is recommended (BIRADs 4 or 5). If a suspicious skin lesion of the nipple is found on examination, punch biopsy should be performed. For example, patients with Paget disease of the breast may present with eczematous changes, erythema, excoriation, or ulceration of the nipple causing bleeding, which may be mischaracterized as nipple discharge. When Paget disease is diagnosed, complete breast imaging is indicated as Paget disease is associated with an underlying malignancy (DICS and/or an invasive cancer) within the breast parenchyma in more than 85% of cases.[44–47]

DISCUSSION—TREATMENT OPTIONS

Physiologic nipple discharge (galactorrhea) is treated based on the most likely underlying cause. Patients on medications associated with galactorrhea (see **Table 1**), most commonly antipsychotics and metoclopramide, may need these altered, changed, or discontinued by the prescribing provider. In cases where the galactorrhea is not overly bothersome to the patient and/or the prescribing physician deems the patient will stay optimally treated on the causative mediation (eg, an antipsychotic), then continuing the medication is appropriate. Referral to an endocrinologist is reasonable if laboratory values (ie, prolactin level or TSH level with reflexive T3/T4) are abnormal and/or if a patient presents with other endocrine symptoms. Patients with galactorrhea but normal

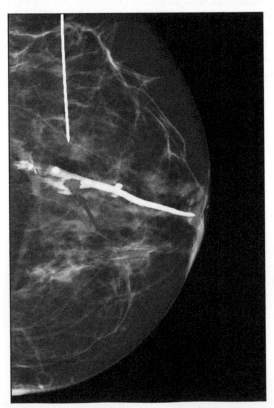

Fig. 3. Mammary galactogram image. Galactogram demonstrating a filling defect (*arrow*) indicating an intraductal lesion. (Original figure courtesy of Jonathan Nguyen, MD.)

prolactin levels can be observed. This is most common in premenopausal women. If the diagnostic workup reveals no findings of concern, patients with galactorrhea can be reassured that this idiopathic phenomenon is benign and most often transient, and they should follow-up in 3 months to ensure resolution.

All women and men with pathologic nipple discharge should be referred to a breast surgeon once the aforementioned diagnostic workup has been completed (see **Fig. 1**).

High-Risk and Malignant Lesions

When diagnostic workup reveals a malignant or high-risk lesion as the underlying cause of a patient's nipple discharge, the patient should be managed per National Comprehensive Cancer Network guidelines.

Benign Lesions

Surgical excision of an intraductal papilloma is warranted if atypia is seen on CNBx, if there is discordance between the CNBx pathologic condition and imaging findings,[48–53] or if the lesion is associated with pathologic nipple discharge[54,55] because these factors increase the risk of it being upstaged to a malignancy on final pathology. Surgical excision is also appropriate if the patient desires resolution of symptoms. In contrast, asymptomatic, radiology-pathology concordant intraductal papillomas less than 1.0 cm in size and without atypia on CNBx are not routinely excised at most centers.[56] Instead, these patients can be offered close clinical and radiological follow-up.[56]

It is important to note that pathologic nipple discharge may sometimes cease after CNBx if the entire lesion or even the majority of it was removed. In this case, consultation between the patient and surgeon will determine next steps—surgical excision versus no further intervention for a benign lesion. For patients who elect no further intervention after cessation of the nipple discharge, short follow-up diagnostic breast imaging (ie, 6 months) is prudent. Finally, if the patient does undergo surgical excision of a benign lesion causing nipple discharge, but the nipple discharge persists, a surgical excision of the discharging duct(s) can be performed. Similarly, patients without an identifiable underlying lesion can be offered a duct excision for the resolution of symptoms and pathologic evaluation of the underlying ductal system (see **Fig. 1**). If a single duct is identified as the source of pathologic discharge, a selective excision of the draining duct may be performed. Alternatively, a complete excision of the retroareolar major duct may be offered, which has the benefit of reducing the risk of recurrent discharge but eliminates the potential for future breastfeeding.[57]

Patients with mammary duct ectasia can be safely observed for symptom resolution. Patients with nonlactational mastitis, with or with an abscess, presenting with purulent nipple discharge should have the underlying infection treated with ultrasound-guided drainage and/or oral antibiotics.

CLINICS CARE POINTS

- Nipple discharge is the third most common breast-related complaint but is rarely the presenting symptom of breast cancer.
- Nipple discharge is categorized as lactational, physiologic, or pathologic.
- Pathologic nipple discharge is typically unilateral, spontaneous, from a single duct, and can range from bloody to serous.
- Patients with pathologic discharge should undergo age-appropriate imaging workup, most often including mammogram and ultrasound. If initial imaging is negative, additional

imaging including MRI, galactogram, and ductoscopy should be considered. Cytologic evaluation of the discharge is not useful.

- All women and men with pathologic nipple discharge should be referred to a breast surgeon for evaluation, treatment, and follow-up.

SUMMARY

Although most patients presenting with nipple discharge have no underlying pathologic condition of concern, the risk of an underlying malignancy warrants thorough evaluation of patients with pathologic nipple discharge. The diagnostic algorithm presented here can be used to distinguish patients with benign, physiologic nipple discharge from those with pathologic nipple discharge. In the setting of pathologic discharge age-appropriate imaging workup and diagnostic evaluation is indicated to assess for an underlying pathologic condition requiring surgical or medical management.

DISCLOSURE

The authors have nothing to disclose.

REFERENCES

1. Hussain AN, Policarpio C, Vincent MT. Evaluating nipple discharge. Obstet Gynecol Surv 2006;61(4):278–83.
2. Newman HF, Klein M, Northrup JD, et al. Nipple discharge. Frequency and pathogenesis in an ambulatory population. N Y State J Med 1983;83(7):928–33.
3. Murad TM, Contesso G, Mouriesse H. Nipple discharge from the breast. Ann Surg 1982;195(3):259–64.
4. Sauter ER, Schlatter L, Lininger J, et al. The association of bloody nipple discharge with breast pathology. Surgery 2004;136(4):780–5.
5. Lee SJ, Trikha S, Moy L, et al. ACR Appropriateness Criteria(®) Evaluation of nipple discharge. J Am Coll Radiol 2017;14(5s):S138–53.
6. Onstad M, Stuckey A. Benign breast disorders. Obstet Gynecol Clin North Am 2013;40(3):459–73.
7. Neville MC, McFadden TB, Forsyth I. Hormonal regulation of mammary differentiation and milk secretion. J Mammary Gland Biol Neoplasia 2002;7(1):49–66.
8. Buhimschi CS. Endocrinology of lactation. Obstet Gynecol Clin North Am 2004; 31(4):963–79, xii.
9. Riordan J, Wambach K. Breastfeeding and human lactation. Jones & Bartlett Learning; 2010.
10. Neville MC, Morton J, Umemura S, et al. The transition from pregnancy to lactation. Pediatr Clin North Am 2001;48(1):35–52.
11. Adriance MC, Inman JL, Petersen OW, et al. Myoepithelial cells: good fences make good neighbors. Breast Cancer Res 2005;7(5):190–7.
12. Molitch ME. Drugs and prolactin. Pituitary 2008;11(2):209–18.
13. Molitch ME. Medication-induced hyperprolactinemia. Mayo Clin Proc 2005;80(8): 1050–7.
14. Coker F, Taylor D. Antidepressant-induced hyperprolactinaemia: incidence, mechanisms and management. CNS Drugs 2010;24(7):563–74.

15. Vargas HI, Vargas MP, Eldrageely K, et al. Outcomes of clinical and surgical assessment of women with pathological nipple discharge. Am Surg 2006;72(2): 124–8.
16. Nelson RS, Hoehn JL. Twenty-year outcome following central duct resection for bloody nipple discharge. Ann Surg 2006;243(4):522–4.
17. Kooistra BW, Wauters C, van de Ven S, et al. The diagnostic value of nipple discharge cytology in 618 consecutive patients. Eur J Surg Oncol 2009;35(6): 573–7.
18. King TA, Carter KM, Bolton JS, et al. A simple approach to nipple discharge. Am Surg 2000;66(10):960–5 [discussion: 965–6].
19. Jardines L. Management of nipple discharge. Am Surg 1996;62(2):119–22.
20. Hamwi MW, Winters R. Mammary Duct Ectasia. StatPearls. StatPearls Publishing-Copyright © 2022. StatPearls Publishing LLC.; 2022.
21. Seltzer MH, Perloff LJ, Kelley RI, et al. The significance of age in patients with nipple discharge. Surg Gynecol Obstet 1970;131(3):519–22.
22. Alcock C, Layer GT. Predicting occult malignancy in nipple discharge. ANZ J Surg 2010;80(9):646–9.
23. Cabioglu N, Hunt KK, Singletary SE, et al. Surgical decision making and factors determining a diagnosis of breast carcinoma in women presenting with nipple discharge. J Am Coll Surg 2003;196(3):354–64.
24. Kalu ON, Chow C, Wheeler A, et al. The diagnostic value of nipple discharge cytology: breast imaging complements predictive value of nipple discharge cytology. J Surg Oncol 15 2012;106(4):381–5.
25. Morrogh M, Park A, Elkin EB, et al. Lessons learned from 416 cases of nipple discharge of the breast. Am J Surg 2010;200(1):73–80.
26. Gülay H, Bora S, Kılıçturgay S, et al. Management of nipple discharge. J Am Coll Surg 1994;178(5):471–4.
27. Klimberg VS. Nipple discharge: more than pathologic. Ann Surg Oncol 2003; 10(2):98–9.
28. Kline TS, Lash SR. The BLEEDING NIPPLE OF PREGNANCY and POSTPARTUM PERIOD; a CYTOLOGIC and HISTOLOGIC STUDY. Acta Cytol 1964;8:336–40.
29. Lafreniere R. Bloody nipple discharge during pregnancy: a rationale for conservative treatment. J Surg Oncol 1990;43(4):228–30.
30. Scott-Conner CE, Schorr SJ. The diagnosis and management of breast problems during pregnancy and lactation. Am J Surg 1995;170(4):401–5.
31. Gray RJ, Pockaj BA, Karstaedt PJ. Navigating murky waters: a modern treatment algorithm for nipple discharge. Am J Surg 2007;194(6):850–4 [discussion: 854–5].
32. Mainiero MB, Lourenco AP, Barke LD, et al. ACR Appropriateness Criteria Evaluation of the Symptomatic Male breast. J Am Coll Radiol 2015;12(7):678–82.
33. Khan SA, Wolfman JA, Segal L, et al. Ductal lavage findings in women with mammographic microcalcifications undergoing biopsy. Ann Surg Oncol 2005; 12(9):689–96.
34. Sickles EA. Galactography and other imaging investigations of nipple discharge. Lancet 2000;356(9242):1622–3.
35. Rissanen T, Reinikainen H, Apaja-Sarkkinen M. Breast sonography in localizing the cause of nipple discharge: comparison with galactography in 52 patients. J Ultrasound Med 2007;26(8):1031–9.
36. Boisserie-Lacroix M, Doutriaux-Dumoulin I, Chopier J, et al. Diagnostic accuracy of breast MRI for patients with suspicious nipple discharge and negative

mammography and ultrasound: a prospective study. Eur Radiol 2021;31(10): 7783–91.

37. Kuhl CK, Schrading S, Bieling HB, et al. MRI for diagnosis of pure ductal carcinoma in situ: a prospective observational study. Lancet 2007;370(9586):485–92.

38. Badan GM, Piato S, Roveda DJ, et al. Predictive values of BI-RADS(®) magnetic resonance imaging (MRI) in the detection of breast ductal carcinoma in situ (DCIS). Eur J Radiol 2016;85(10):1701–7.

39. Ballesio L, Maggi C, Savelli S, et al. Role of breast magnetic resonance imaging (MRI) in patients with unilateral nipple discharge: preliminary study. Radiol Med 2008;113(2):249–64.

40. Berger N, Luparia A, Di Leo G, et al. Diagnostic Performance of MRI versus galactography in women with pathologic nipple discharge: a Systematic review and meta-analysis. AJR Am J Roentgenol 2017;209(2):465–71.

41. Morrogh M, Morris EA, Liberman L, et al. The predictive value of ductography and magnetic resonance imaging in the management of nipple discharge. Ann Surg Oncol 2007;14(12):3369–77.

42. Adepoju LJ, Chun J, El-Tamer M, et al. The value of clinical characteristics and breast-imaging studies in predicting a histopathologic diagnosis of cancer or high-risk lesion in patients with spontaneous nipple discharge. Am J Surg 2005;190(4):644–6.

43. Cardenosa G, Doudna C, Eklund GW. Ductography of the breast: technique and findings. AJR Am J Roentgenol 1994;162(5):1081–7.

44. Chen CY, Sun LM, Anderson BO. Paget disease of the breast: changing patterns of incidence, clinical presentation, and treatment in the U.S. Cancer 2006;107(7): 1448–58.

45. Ikeda DM, Helvie MA, Frank TS, et al. Paget disease of the nipple: radiologic-pathologic correlation. Radiology 1993;189(1):89–94.

46. Lloyd J, Flanagan AM. Mammary and extramammary Paget's disease. J Clin Pathol 2000;53(10):742–9.

47. Dalberg K, Hellborg H, Wärnberg F. Paget's disease of the nipple in a population based cohort. Breast Cancer Res Treat 2008;111(2):313–9.

48. Lewis JT, Hartmann LC, Vierkant RA, et al. An analysis of breast cancer risk in women with single, multiple, and atypical papilloma. Am J Surg Pathol 2006; 30(6):665–72.

49. Valdes EK, Feldman SM, Boolbol SK. Papillary lesions: a review of the literature. Ann Surg Oncol 2007;14(3):1009–13.

50. Mercado CL, Hamele-Bena D, Oken SM, et al. Papillary lesions of the breast at percutaneous core-needle biopsy. Radiology 2006;238(3):801–8.

51. Sydnor MK, Wilson JD, Hijaz TA, et al. Underestimation of the presence of breast carcinoma in papillary lesions initially diagnosed at core-needle biopsy. Radiology 2007;242(1):58–62.

52. Ahmadiyeh N, Stoleru MA, Raza S, et al. Management of intraductal papillomas of the breast: an analysis of 129 cases and their outcome. Ann Surg Oncol 2009; 16(8):2264–9.

53. Wen X, Cheng W. Nonmalignant breast papillary lesions at core-needle biopsy: a meta-analysis of underestimation and influencing factors. Ann Surg Oncol 2013; 20(1):94–101.

54. Han SH, Kim M, Chung YR, et al. Benign intraductal papilloma without atypia on core needle biopsy has a Low rate of Upgrading to malignancy after Excision. J Breast Cancer 2018;21(1):80–6.

55. Ahn SK, Han W, Moon HG, et al. Management of benign papilloma without atypia diagnosed at ultrasound-guided core needle biopsy: Scoring system for predicting malignancy. Eur J Surg Oncol 2018;44(1):53–8.
56. Surgeons" ASoB. Consensus guideline on concordance assessment of image-guided breast biopsies and management of borderline or high-risk lesions. Available at: https://www.breastsurgeons.org/docs/statements/Consensus-Guideline-on-Concordance-Assessment-of-Image-Guided-Breast-Biopsies.pdf.
57. Fuhrman GM, King TA. Multidisciplinary breast management. Surg Clin North Am 2013;93(2):xvii–xviii.

Management of Cystic Conditions

Holly Ortman, MD, James Abdo, MD*, Rachel Tillman, MD, Anna Seydel, MD

KEYWORDS

- Benign breast disease • Fibrocystic change • Cystic conditions • Simple cyst
- Complex cyst • Complicated cyst

KEY POINTS

- Asymptomatic simple cysts do not need intervention.
- Fibrocystic condition is common and broadly encompasses the response of normal breast tissue to hormonal changes.
- Cysts that rapidly refill or masses that persist after aspiration require core needle biopsy
- Complicated and complex cysts have a risk of malignancy and should undergo biopsy

INTRODUCTION

Breast cysts are the most common nonproliferative disorder of the breast. Up to one-third of women aged 30 to 50 years have cysts in their breasts. Despite its prevalence, there is marked heterogeneity in how breast cysts are managed in clinical practice. The widespread use of screening radiologic modalities has increased the number of nonpalpable, asymptomatic breast lesions being diagnosed each year and has placed a large portion of the diagnosis and subsequent management on the radiologist. However, careful explanation and examination remain the responsibility of the breast clinician. In the context of fibrocystic change, the management of patients with simple, complicated, and complex cysts is discussed. The information is organized for easy reference for the surgeon caring for women with benign cystic conditions of the breast. A practical discussion has also been included at the end of the article for surgeons taking care of women with benign cystic conditions of the breast.

FIBROCYSTIC CHANGES

Fibrocystic changes is a nonspecific term that refers to responses of breast tissue to normal hormonal changes throughout a woman's life. These changes do not have

Department of Surgery, Marshfield Medical Center, 1000 N. Oak Avenue, Marshfield, WI 54449, USA
* Corresponding author. Abdo.James@marshfieldclinic.org
E-mail address: Abdo.James@marshfieldclinic.org

Surg Clin N Am 102 (2022) 1089–1102
https://doi.org/10.1016/j.suc.2022.07.004
0039-6109/22/© 2022 Elsevier Inc. All rights reserved.

malignant potential. Some definitions limit fibrocystic changes to nonproliferative histologic descriptions,[1] whereas others use it interchangeably with benign epithelial lesions. Some others even use this term to encompass all benign breast disease. Breast pathologists have progressed to accurately reporting the histologic variations of benign changes and are no longer using the umbrella term, *fibrocystic changes*. This progress has led to confusion for breast clinicians.[2,3] Although the histopathology may be diverse, the clinical correlation to both symptoms and concern for malignancy have been identified and are important to understand.[3]

Women with fibrocystic changes classically present with "lumpy bumpy" breasts, with diffuse, palpable densities often in large areas of the breast that are sometimes tender. These patients often present with cyclic pain, tenderness, or palpable masses. Cystic conditions of the breast most commonly present in the third decade, peak in the fourth decade, and dramatically decrease in incidence after menopause. Some report these changes are evident in up to 60% of women examined clinically and up to 90% of women in histopathologic studies.[4] Cystic change is caused by alteration of lobules, starting with dilation and then coalescence of the ductules with unfolding or involution of the terminal duct lobular units (TLDUs) in response to cyclic hormonal changes.[5] Smaller cysts often then coalesce to form larger cysts lined by atrophic epithelium or metaplastic apocrine cells. These benign cysts frequently rupture and release secretory material into the adjacent stroma resulting in chronic inflammation contributing to the palpable nodularity of the breast.[1,2] Simple cysts and apocrine cysts are nonproliferative and are often found incidentally in specimens removed or biopsied for other indications. Cysts, however, can also be identified microscopically alongside proliferative changes with or without atypia. Cysts will also frequently have calcifications formed from secretory debris. These clustered calcifications along with the density of surrounding fibrosis may be radiologically suspicious and difficult to differentiate from malignant disease[6] (**Figs. 1** and **2**).

Microscopically, fibrocystic changes that include cysts can be grouped based on risk stratification. Owing to the variety of histologic variations seen with benign fibrocystic change, DuPont and Page proposed a classification system based on risk of malignancy and presence of atypia. Fibrocystic changes are classified as nonproliferative, proliferative without atypia, and proliferative with atypia (atypical hyperplasia), each with its own unique reported risk of developing breast cancer[7,8] (**Table 1**).

As with any patient being seen for breast pathologic condition, consideration of risk factors for breast cancer is an essential aspect of evaluation and is often one of the greatest concerns of those presenting with symptoms or a newly identified mass. Although these relative risks are associated with the histologic findings on biopsy, the patient's age at the time of biopsy and her family history of breast cancer also play a role in determining a woman's risk of breast cancer after a diagnosis of benign breast disease. Of note, about 70% of biopsies identifying benign breast disease are nonproliferative lesions with no increased risk of cancer.[7]

APOCRINE-LINED CYSTS

Apocrine change, including apocrine-lined cysts, is a nonproliferative disorder of the breast reflecting involution of tissue responsive to normal hormonal fluctuations. In fibrocystic change, an apocrine metaplastic cell layer lines the cystically dilated acini, which are filled with fluid and often contain calcified particles. Microscopically, a single epithelial cell layer is identified that shows apocrine changes because it has been disrupted by this process of obstruction. Apocrine metaplasia is present in the epithelial lining of the cysts. The presence of apocrine metaplasia or the findings of an apocrine-

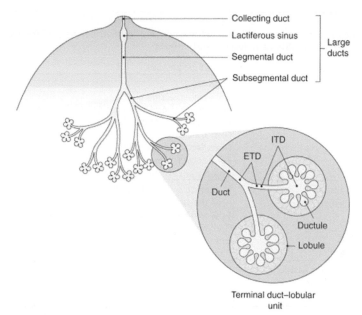

Fig. 1. The structure of terminal duct-lobular units. Laura C. Collins, Breat, in J. R. Goldblum, L. W. Lamps, J. K. McKenney, J. L. Myers, L. V. Ackerman, and J. Rosai, Rosai and Ackerman's surgical pathology. 2018. Accessed: Feb. 24, 2022.

lined cyst on final pathology of an excised specimen or core needle biopsy (CNB) is of no additional clinical significance and does not confer an added breast cancer risk (**Fig. 3**).

SIMPLE CYST

A simple cyst is a round, well-circumscribed structure with thin walls. Simple cysts are epithelium lined and fluid filled. Simple cysts are derived from a TLDU whose epithelial lining is either flattened or absent.[9] The defining characteristics of simple cysts on ultrasonography include the presence of posterior acoustical enhancement and the

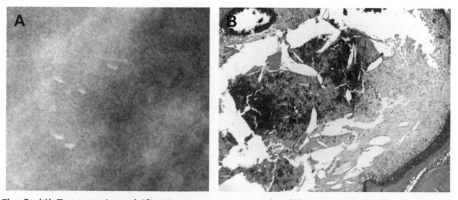

Fig. 2. (A) Teacup microcalcification on mammography. (B) Microcystic "milk of calcium" lamellar calcifications, which may form sediment on the floor of the cyst to produce the teacup calcification pattern.[5]

Table 1
[9]Relative risk of cancer in patients found to have nonproliferative lesions, proliferative lesions without atypia, and proliferative lesions with atypia

Histologic Category	Histologic Lesions	Relative Risk
Nonproliferative lesions	Cysts Papillary apocrine change Epithelial-related calcifications Mild epithelial hyperplasia Ductal ectasia Nonsclerosing adenosis Periductal fibrosis Columnar cell change	1
Proliferative lesions without atypia	Moderate or florid ductal hyperplasia of the usual type Sclerosing adenosis Radial scar Intraductal papilloma Papillomatosis	1.3–1.9
Proliferative lesions with atypia (atypical hyperplasia)	Atypical ductal hyperplasia Atypical lobular hyperplasia	3.9–13.0

Adapted from M. Guray and A. A. Sahin, "Benign breast diseases: classification, diagnosis, and management," The Oncologist, vol. 11, no. 5, pp. 435–449, May 2006, https://doi.org/10.1634/theoncologist.11-5-435.

absence of internal echoes and solid components. Septa are present in some cases of simple cysts; however, the septa must be less than 0.5 mm in thickness to maintain the classification of a simple cyst. Cysts larger than 3 mm may be palpable and prompt diagnostic imaging. In addition to individual cysts, clustered microcysts may be seen on ultrasound examination. Clustered microcysts represent a subset of simple cysts and are defined as numerous simple anechoic cysts, each smaller than 2 to 3 mm, without discrete solid components. Simple cysts are found in as many as one-third of women aged 35 to 50 years. Simple cysts are hormone-sensitive, which corresponds to the peak incidence in premenopausal women. Cysts are also seen in postmenopausal women on hormone therapy at a frequency higher than postmenopausal women not on hormonal therapy.

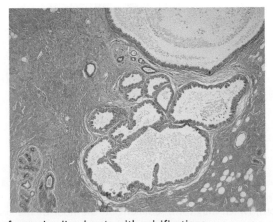

Fig. 3. Pathology of apocrine-lined cysts with calcifications.

Patients with simple cysts may present to the clinic with a palpable mass, with or without associated symptoms. Associated symptoms may include erythema, skin changes over the cyst, pain (both cyclical and non-cyclical) and induration around the area, nipple inversion, nipple discharge.

For these patients, physical examination, although critical in the evaluation of a new breast mass, is a poor diagnostic tool because it is almost impossible to discern a cyst from a solid mass without imaging. It is no longer standard of care to proceed with a blind fine-needle aspiration (FNA) at the bedside to check for fluid in a patient presenting with a palpable mass. Diagnostic imaging is determined by the patient's age, with bilateral diagnostic mammogram often recommended in addition to focused ultrasonography for patients older than 30 years.[10] For patients younger than 30 years, an ultrasonography is often the only diagnostic modality indicated. Mammography is reserved for this patient population if the physician has concerns for malignancy. For patients who are confirmed to have a simple cyst on imaging, aspiration is recommended at any age if symptoms are present or if there is documented rapid increase in size of the cyst. Cyst fluid that is straw-colored, opaque, or green can be discarded. Aspiration can be performed at the bedside with or without ultrasonographic guidance, but it is best tolerated using ultrasonography as a guide, which allows the physician to visualize collapse of the cyst and complete aspiration of the fluid. If the aspirate appears purulent, it should be sent for microbiologic analysis with cultures and antibiotic sensitivity. Bloody aspirate should be sent for cytology to rule out malignancy. If the cyst does not fully collapse after aspiration, a CNB can be performed of the remaining cyst wall to obtain tissue diagnosis.[11] After aspiration, if full collapse is demonstrated and the patient's symptoms improve, the patient may resume annual screening if age appropriate.

To summarize, no further evaluation is needed for patients who are found on screening mammogram to have a mass that is confirmed on diagnostic imaging to be a simple cyst. To be regarded as a simple cyst, a breast mass must meet 3 criteria on ultrasonography—a sharp margin with an abrupt transition between the mass and surrounding tissue, anechoic without internal echoes, and a column of increased echogenicity deep to the mass (posterior acoustic enhancement). Breast masses meeting these criteria are considered simple cysts, and are Breast Imaging Reporting and Data System (BI-RADS) 2: Benign (**Table 2**). Ultrasonography has 98% accuracy for diagnosing simple cysts; no additional follow-up is indicated. There is no indication to obtain tissue diagnosis for patients who present with an asymptomatic breast mass that is confirmed to be a simple cyst on imaging. The American Society of Breast Surgeons has stated "Don't routinely drain non-painful fluid-filled breast cysts" in their Choosing Wisely campaign, which aims to educate both patients and physicians in managing breast disease in an effort to eliminate unnecessary procedures and standardize management[12] (**Fig. 4**).

With a diagnostic mammogram, a simple cyst (see earlier) can be seen as a well-circumscribed mass. A common finding is its low density—normal fibroglandular tissue and parenchymal features can be seen through the mass. After obtaining a mammogram, follow-up imaging with ultrasonography is recommended to further evaluate the characteristics of the lesion.

COMPLICATED CYST

Complicated cysts differ from simple cysts only with regard to internal echoes. Complicated cysts are thin-walled cysts with homogeneous hypoechoic material present inside. The low-level internal echoes are created from debris in the cyst, likely

BI-RADS Category	Definition	Likelihood of Malignancy	Management Recommendation
	Table 2 **American College of Radiology Breast Imaging Reporting and Data System Code assessment categories[13]**		
0	Incomplete - Need Additional Imaging Evaluation and/or Prior Mammograms for Comparison	N/A	Recall for additional imaging and/or comparison with prior examination(s)
1	Negative	Essentially 0%	Routine mammography screening
2	Benign	Essentially 0%	Routine mammography screening
3	Probably benign a	>0% but ≤2%	Short-interval (6-month) follow-up or continued surveillance mammography
4	Suspicious	>2% but <95%	Tissue diagnosis
4A	Low suspicion for malignancy	>2% to ≤10%	Tissue diagnosis
4B	Moderate suspicion for malignancy	>10% to ≤50%	Tissue diagnosis
4C	High suspicion for malignancy	>50% to <95%	Tissue diagnosis
5	Highly suggestive of malignancy	≥95%	Tissue diagnosis
6	Known biopsy-proven malignancy	N/A	Surgical excision when clinically appropriate

Abbreviations: BI-RADS, Breast Imaging Reporting and Data System; N/A, not applicable.

proteins from cell turnover, hemorrhage, or purulence. The internal echoes may also change shape with a change in patient positioning and can demonstrate fluid levels. Like a simple cyst, a complicated cyst does not have thick walls, thick septa, or vascular flow (**Fig. 5**).

Complicated cysts are defined on ultrasonography and are described as a circumscribed, oval mass that is in parallel orientation and contains low-level echoes throughout the mass. There is no solid component present, nor are there septations or a thick outer wall.[14] Patients may be symptomatic or asymptomatic on presentation. Cystic diseases of the breast are relatively common and are often incidentally found on screening mammography. There is ongoing debate regarding management of findings of complicated cysts in both radiology and surgery, because these cysts have most, but not all, features one would find in a simple cyst. FNA may be used to help differentiate cystic from solid masses as well as determine the contents of the cyst. If the FNA is performed via ultrasonography, resolution of the cyst following aspiration will also aid in diagnosis and may determine the success of the therapeutic aspiration.

Aspiration of symptomatic or nonsimple palpable cysts is recommended by the National Comprehensive Cancer Network guidelines; however, recent studies have brought this into question due to the low cancer rate in complicated cysts. Breast cancer found in complicated cyst as defined by ultrasonography is quite rare (approximately 0.4%). Because of this exceedingly low rate of malignancy, discussions in

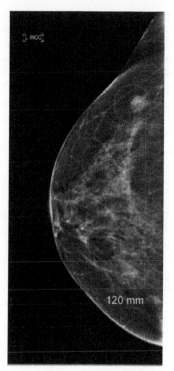

Fig. 4. Ultrasonographic and mammographic findings of simple cysts. Note the thin wall, lack of internal debris, and posterior acoustic enhancement seen on ultrasonography.

2019 have entertained reclassification of complicated cysts as probably benign (BI-RADS 3), which would require only follow-up instead of FNA or biopsy.[15,16] This reclassification has not yet translated into formal guidelines. Currently, patients who do not undergo biopsy are referred for short-term follow-up at 6 or 12 months. In this population, however, it has been found that they have a lower compliance rate than women who are recommended to undergo aspiration or CNB.[17] Of those that

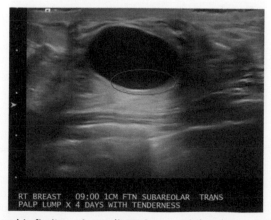

Fig. 5. Ultrasonographic finding of complicated cyst with low-level internal echoes.

do undergo aspiration and nonbloody fluid is sent for cytology, the majority are benign. Approximately half of the lesions that are aspirated are discarded because they contain typical cyst fluid and do not require cytology. In a study to evaluate whether or not aspiration of fluid from complicated cysts was necessary to rule out malignancy, Daly and colleagues[17] found that only 1 of 184 lesions with typical cyst fluid contained atypia and fibrocystic changes were found on excision. One of 22 bloody aspirates contained atypia and atypical lobular hyperplasia.[17] In this same study, 1 of 243 patients was diagnosed with invasive cancer when a solid mass persisted after aspiration and collapse of 2 adjacent complicated cysts. These studies support the discussion of reclassifying complicated cysts to short-interval follow-up without need for FNA.

COMPLEX CYST

Complex cysts are thick-walled (>0.5 mm) structures with or without septa measuring greater than 0.5 mm in thickness. The borders may be irregular due to the mixed characteristics of the cyst itself and can be macrolobulated or microlobulated. These cysts typically consist of a mix of cystic and solid components and may lack posterior wall enhancement on ultrasonography (**Figs. 6** and **7**).

Additional ultrasonographic findings may reveal anechoic and echogenic components. According to Berg and colleagues, complex cysts can be categorized into 4 categories based on ultrasonographic appearance (**Table 3**).

Complex breast cysts, defined by ultrasound criteria, have a 23% to 31%[18] risk of malignancy and are BI-RADS category 4 or 5. The patient may be asymptomatic or have nonspecific symptoms including unilateral pain, tenderness, cyclical pain, and palpable mass. A breast cyst that acutely enlarges may cause sudden onset of severe unilateral localized breast pain. On examination, the patient may have a palpable mass, but there is not a physical examination characteristic or presenting symptom that is specific to complex breast cysts, so it is indistinguishable from malignancy without imaging and biopsy.

CYST WITH PAPILLARY COMPONENT

Papillary lesions of the breast represent a spectrum of disease ranging from benign to atypical to malignant and can be identified as a complex cyst with solid elements.

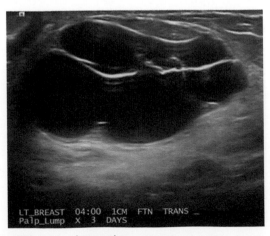

Fig. 6. Complex cyst with internal septations present.

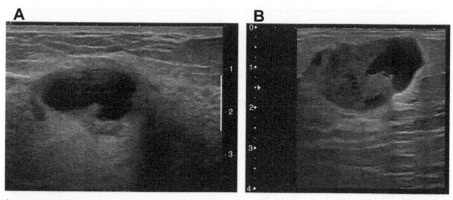

Fig. 7. Complex cystic and solid masses in 2 different patients. These were managed with fluid aspiration and core biopsy of the solid component. Histopathology of (*A*) chronic inflammation and fat necrosis, consistent with ruptured duct. Histopathology of (*B*) intracystic papillary carcinoma.

Considering the limitation of FNA, findings are not completely specific so the accuracy of discriminating between benign and malignant papillary lesions is poor. In a study by He and colleagues,[19] FNA assisted in evaluation of papillary lesions and was able to prevent false-negative results on simultaneous CNB, so when these were performed in combination, the diagnosis was more specific, lending to correct clinical management. Similar to papillary, there are other cystic breast lesions that may have a variety of findings on ultrasonography including complex cyst with solid components and may be benign, atypical, or malignant.

There are multiple benign (**Table 4**)[18] and malignant conditions that may result in a complex cyst on ultrasonography, and the management varies based on the findings.

Fluid component is sent for cytology, rather than being discarded as in simple cysts. FNA and CNB should be performed in the same session if a solid component is present.[20] When there is a known solid component, core biopsies should be performed initially. A postbiopsy marker should always be placed on completion of the biopsy.[21] As described in Youk and colleagues,[20] when the biopsy results are concordant with the imaging findings, follow-up should be performed in 6 months, before resuming routine monitoring. In a patient with a high-risk lesion, surgical excision should be considered because these lesions have been shown to have an increased rate of malignancy. When the biopsy is discordant with the ultrasonographic findings, then either repeat biopsy or surgical excision should be discussed with the patient.

Table 3 Complex cyst characteristics		
Type	**Description**	**PPV for Malignancy**
Type I	Masses with a thick wall (>0.5 mm) or thick septa (>0.5 mm)	7.1%
Type II	Masses of an intracystic type with one or more discrete solid mural lesions within a cyst	16.7%
Type III	Masses containing mixed cystic and solid components with the cystic portion occupying at least 50% of the mass	61.1%
Type IV	Masses that were predominantly (at least 50%) solid with eccentric or central cystic foci	44.8%

Abbreviation: PPV, positive predictive value.

Table 4
Benign and malignant cystic conditions, imaging findings, and management

Benign	Ultrasonographic/Clinical Findings	Biopsy	Follow-up
Inflammatory cysts/ruptured	Thick wall or internal septum >0.5 mm		
Apocrine metaplasia and fibrocystic mastopathy	Grouping of microcysts. Thick wall or internal septum >0.5 mm	FNA adequate	
Fat necrosis	Thick wall, connection to scar on skin, no hyperemia. Thick wall or internal septum >0.5 mm		
Hematoma/seroma/lymphocele	Recent trauma/surgery. Thick wall or internal septum >0.5 mm		Ultrasonography repeat in 4–6 mo
Breast abscess	Fever, pain, local hyperemia, inflammatory skin changes. Thick wall or internal septum >0.5 mm	FNA adequate	
Juvenile papillomatosis	Nodular image with multiple cysts. Thick wall or internal septum >0.5 mm		Surgically ablated – high risk lesion
Cystic breast lymphangioma	Multiloculated, slow growing. Thick wall or internal septum >0.5 mm	FNA adequate	Surgical ablation due to size
Modified cysts ± mobile debris	Predominantly cystic complex masses		
Posttherapeutic fat necrosis	Predominantly cystic complex mass. History of procedure	Correlation between history, mammogram, and ultrasound may negate need for biopsy	
Galactocele	Complex mass, several fluid/fluid levels. Context of breast feeding		

Papillary lesions (benign and atypical)	Nipple discharge. Intralesional flow in vascular stalk	Biopsy	Surgical ablation recommended to analyze entire lesion
Fibrocystic mastopathy	Predominantly solid complex masses		
Complex fibroadenomas	Predominantly solid complex mass. Cysts >3 mm, adenosis, epithelial calcifications, apocrine metaplasia		
Phyllodes tumor	Cystic slits		Surgical ablation to analyze entire lesion

GENERAL PRINCIPLES

For surgeons who see patients with benign breast disease, a good working relationship with a trusted pathologist and radiologist is paramount. Patients are often referred to the breast clinic directly from the radiology department with imaging findings suggestive of a benign cause and inconclusive pathology results with questions on how best to proceed. Diagnostic uncertainty remains an indication for excision of benign disease, and the decision to proceed to the operating room is solely between the surgeon and the patient. Concordance assessment of the histology, imaging, and clinical findings determines further management and is ultimately the responsibility of the surgeon. Discordance occurs when a breast CNB shows benign histology, whereas the clinical or imaging findings are suspicious for malignancy.[22,23] When a biopsy result is discordant, the decision about how best to obtain additional tissue and whether the patient is a candidate to proceed with further intervention is made by the surgeon who is best able to assess the risk to the patient.

Other than diagnostic uncertainty, operative intervention for patients with benign cystic conditions of the breast is reserved for complications from aspiration. Rarely, patients will develop complications of infection, abscess, or fistula formation as a result of repeat aspiration. In these rare instances, surgical principles of soft tissue infection apply. In addition, in a busy breast practice, it is common to have patients referred urgently from their primary care physician for a painful breast cyst that has been confirmed by imaging evaluation with findings of a sebaceous cyst on clinical examination.

The goal of an operation for benign cystic disease is to either alleviate symptoms or obtain an adequate sample for accurate tissue diagnosis. Regardless of the localization technique or placement of incision, the final pathology must include the previous biopsy site and a specimen radiograph confirming the clip should be obtained. Although most clips are not visible or palpable at the time of excisional biopsy, biopsy site changes, when intraoperatively present, can guide the extent of excision. Patients and surgeons have a higher standard for final cosmetic appearance of the breast when operating for benign disease and are less tolerant of parenchymal defects than with a cancer operation. That said, "the right amount" of tissue needs to be removed to assure an accurate diagnosis. During an operation for benign disease, it is common to encounter fluid-filled, dilated ducts and palpable changes within the breast. Taking time to examine the breast tissue in the operating room and to remove additional abnormal breast tissue around the targeted benign lesion can provide important information about the patient's underlying risk and subsequent management.

If the targeted clip is not present on specimen radiograph, the surgeon must decide whether to continue to excise more breast tissue (without a preoperative diagnosis of cancer), or close the defect and wait for pathology. Fortunately this is a rare occurrence and the options of how best to proceed include blindly excising surrounding tissue, searching for the clip on and around the operative field, proceeding with sterile imaging of the patient on the table, or waiting for final pathology. The flowchart of decision making during an operation for benign disease must include how to proceed if the localizing system fails or the targeted lesion is not confirmed on specimen radiograph.

SUMMARY

Benign cystic conditions of the breast are common and represent a broad category of disorders each presenting with unique clinical symptoms, imaging results, and pathologic findings. Understanding the cause and natural history of this spectrum of benign entities will help minimize unnecessary procedures and maximize outcomes for patients.

CLINICS CARE POINTS

- Simple cysts, clusters of simple microcysts, and a majority of complicated cysts are considered BI-RADS 2 (benign) and do not require biopsy or short term follow up. Complicated cysts may, at times, be BI-RADS 3 (probably benign) and should undergo short term follow up and imaging (six month interval). Complex cysts are BI-RADS 4 or 5 (suspicious or highly suggestive of malignancy) and require a biopsy (ultrasound-guided core needle biopsy).

- Symptomatic simple cysts (appear infected, inflamed, or painful) may be aspirated under ultrasound-guidance to ensure complete cyst collapse. Only frankly bloody aspirate should be further studied via culture and cytology. Aspirate that is green, yellow, or clear is considered benign.

- Complete cyst collapse after aspiration is considered concordant. If there is incomplete collapse, core needle biopsy should be performed.

- When performing a biopsy of a breast lesion (including cysts), it is imperative that a marker be left to potentially guide surgical management pending pathology results. Aspirated cysts may be unable to be later identified after the initial aspiration and biopsy.

DISCLOSURE

The authors do not have any relevant financial interest or other relationship(s) with a commercial entity producing health-care related product and/or services.

REFERENCES

1. Kumar V, Abbas A, Aster J, editors. Robbins & Cotran pathologic basis of disease. 10th edition. Philadelphia (PA): Elsevier; 2021.
2. Goldblum JR, Lamps LW, McKenney JK, et al. Rosai and Ackerman's surgical pathology 2018. Available at: https://www.clinicalkey.com/dura/browse/bookChapter/3-s2.0-C20131134983. Accessed February 24, 2022.
3. Bland K. The breast: Comprehensive management of benign and malignant diseases. Philadelphia (PA): Elsevier; 2018.
4. Meisner ALW, Houman Fekrazad M, Royce ME. Breast Disease: Benign and Malignant. Med Clin North Am 2008;92(5):1115–41. https://doi.org/10.1016/j.mcna.2008.04.003.
5. Dabbs DJ, editor. Breast pathology. 2nd edition. Philadelphia (PA): Elsevier; 2017.
6. Klatt EC, Robbins SL. Robbins and Cotran atlas of pathology 2021. Available at: http://www.vlebooks.com/vleweb/product/openreader?id=none&isbn=9780323640190. Accessed February 24, 2022.
7. Hartmann LC, Sellers TA, Frost MH, et al. Benign Breast Disease and the Risk of Breast Cancer. N Engl J Med 2005;353(3):229–37.
8. Santen RJ, Mansel R. Benign Breast Disorders. N Engl J Med 2005;353(3):275–85.
9. Guray M, Sahin AA. Benign breast diseases: classification, diagnosis, and management. Oncologist 2006;11(5):435–49.
10. Berg WA, Sechtin AG, Marques H, et al. Cystic breast masses and the ACRIN 6666 experience. Radiol Clin North Am 2010;48(5):931–87.
11. Brennan M, Houssami N, French J. Management of benign breast conditions. Part 3–Other breast problems. Aust Fam Physician 2005;34(5):353–5.

12. Non-painful fluid-filled breast cysts | Choosing Wisely," Jan. 08. Available at: https://www.choosingwisely.org/clinician-lists/asbrs-benign-breast-disease-draining-non-painful-fluid-filled-breasts-cysts/. Accessed February 28, 2022.

13. American College of Radiology and BI-RADS Committee, ACR BI-RADS atlas breast imaging and reporting data system. 2013.

14. Mercado CL. BI-RADS update. Radiol Clin North Am 2014;52(3):481–7.

15. Ataya D, Niell BL. Complicated Cysts: Should Management Depend Upon Age? Acad Radiol 2019;26(7):907–8.

16. Aujero MP, Tirada N, Khorjekar G. Asymptomatic Complicated Cysts in Postmenopausal Women: Is Tissue Sampling Unnecessarily High? Acad Radiol 2019; 26(7):900–6.

17. Daly CP, Bailey JE, Klein KA, et al. Complicated breast cysts on sonography: is aspiration necessary to exclude malignancy? Acad Radiol 2008;15(5):610–7.

18. Athanasiou A, Aubert E, Vincent Salomon A, et al. Complex cystic breast masses in ultrasound examination. Diagn Interv Imaging 2014;95(2):169–79.

19. He X, Wang Y, Nam G, et al. A 10 year retrospective review of fine needle aspiration cytology of cystic lesions of the breast with emphasis on papillary cystic lesions. Diagn Cytopathol 2019;47(5):400–3.

20. Youk JH, Kim E-K, Kim MJ, et al. Missed breast cancers at US-guided core needle biopsy: how to reduce them. Radiogr Rev Publ Radiol Soc N Am Inc 2007; 27(1):79–94.

21. Plantade R. Interventional radiology: the corner-stone of breast management. Diagn Interv Imaging 2013;94(6):575–91.

22. "Consensus Guideline on Concordance Assessment of Image-Guided Breast Biopsies and Management of Borderline or High-Risk Lesions," p. 12.

23. Ikeda DM, Miyake KK. Breast imaging. 3rd edition. St Louis (MO): Elsevier; 2017.

Management of Mastitis, Abscess, and Fistula

Howard C. Snider, MD

KEYWORDS

- Subareolar abscess • Subareolar fistula • Zuska's disease • Periductal mastitis
- Squamous metaplasia

KEY POINTS

- Unlike lactational abscesses and nonlactational peripheral breast abscesses, subareolar abscesses tend to recur or develop duct-cutaneous fistulae.
- Smoking and/or congenitally cleft nipples lead to squamous metaplasia in terminal lactiferous ducts.
- Squamous cells secrete keratin which fills and plugs the terminal ducts leading to subareolar infection.
- Successful treatment of recurrent periductal mastitis or Zuska's disease (ZD) requires excision of the obstructed terminal ducts in the nipple.

INTRODUCTION

There are many breast conditions that produce pain or inflammation, not all of which involve infection. Mastalgia, granulomatous mastitis, and other noninfectious mastopathies are covered elsewhere in this publication. Breast infections are broadly categorized as either lactational or nonlactational, and the former are also covered in a different section. The focus of this article is on nonlactational breast infections which are generally subdivided into subareolar and peripheral breast infections because there are significant differences in the etiology and clinical course of each. Peripheral abscesses behave like abscesses in other parts of the body[1] and usually do not recur after treatment with antibiotics, aspiration, or incision and drainage. Unlike peripheral breast and other soft tissue abscesses, infections in the subareolar region have a much higher tendency to recur.

SUBAREOLAR ABSCESSES AND FISTULAE
Background

Few conditions have been more exasperating to patients and challenging to surgeons than chronic subareolar abscesses and fistulae. The fistulous condition was reported

The author has nothing to disclose.
524 Twelve Oaks, Pike Road, Alabama, AL 36064, USA
E-mail address: hsnidermd@gmail.com

Surg Clin N Am 102 (2022) 1103–1116
https://doi.org/10.1016/j.suc.2022.06.007
0039-6109/22/© 2022 Elsevier Inc. All rights reserved.

in 1951 as a distinct clinical entity separate from abscesses elsewhere in the breast by Zuska, Crile, and Ayers.[2] Joseph Zuska was George Crile's resident at the Cleveland Clinic, and his wife suffered from bilateral breast fistulae, stimulating his interest in the condition.[3] Following his wife's operation at the Cleveland Clinic, Zuska's interest in the disease continued at the National Naval Medical Center where 4 additional patients were operated upon before the publication. The authors were prescient in recognizing the underlying problem and the *sine qua non* for successful treatment. "Local excision of the sinus tract and its indurated base without removal or incision of the terminal portion of the involved duct results in recurrence of the abscess or in persistence of the drainage," they wrote. "The most effective treatment of fistulas of lactiferous ducts is excision of the terminal portion of the involved mammary duct along with the indurated base of the sinus."

Although several articles were published in the next few years that cited the work of Zuska, and colleagues,[4–6] the newly described entity did not enjoy widespread dissemination in the surgical community. Two decades later, George Crile, frustrated because surgical textbooks were still not including the topic and students were not being taught about it, suggested the catchy eponym Zuska's disease (ZD) in hopes that the condition would become more widely recognized, and proper treatment would be implemented by surgeons.[7] The suggestion caught on, and the condition is now commonly referred to by its eponym. Crile also suggested an alternative name, SMOLD, for squamous metaplasia of lactiferous ducts, and that name is also occasionally used to describe the same clinical entity.

The terminology in the literature has been confusing, and various terms including periductal mastitis, duct ectasia, varicocele tumor, plasma cell mastitis, comedomastitis, mastitis obliterans, and secretory disease of the breast have been used to describe various conditions that involve subareolar ducts.[8] In 1989, Dixon postulated that all of those names, including periductal mastitis and duct ectasia, referred to different stages of the same disease process. However, after prospectively evaluating 14,225 patients, Dixon, and colleagues,[9] concluded that the 2 conditions were separate, unrelated entities. Dixon defines periductal mastitis as patients who have a periareolar inflammatory mass, a nonlactational subareolar abscess, or a mammary duct fistula. Although he did not evaluate patients for squamous metaplasia, what he calls periductal mastitis is certainly the same as ZD. This perplexing condition affords the opportunity for surgeons to become one more in a long list of physicians who have failed to solve the patient's problem or to earn the unending gratitude of the patient by recognizing the underlying pathogenesis and curing her with an appropriate operation.

Presentation

Although patients with subareolar abscesses and fistulae have been reported from as young as 14[3,10,11] to as old as 79[12] years and to involve men[13–15] as well as women, the typical presentation is a woman in her thirties. Most commonly she will have either a history of chronic smoking,[16–19] a congenital cleft in the central portion of the nipple,[5,6,12,20,21] or both. If the patient is seen early in the course of the disease, she may have only pain and erythema in the peri-areolar region, with or without a palpable mass. As the disease progresses, an abscess usually develops and is almost always located at the border of the areola (**Fig. 1**). If an abscess has previously drained spontaneously or has been incised, an intermittently draining fistulous opening might be present at the border of the areola (**Fig. 2**). Commonly, exasperated patients present after having had multiple drainage procedures and operations that have failed to correct the underlying problem. Lambert, and colleagues,[22] reported an average of 5 prior subareolar abscesses in 37 patients before being seen by them. One patient had

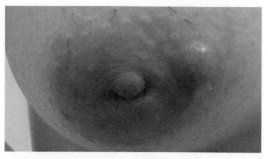

Fig. 1. Subareolar abscess Note the abscess is pointing at the border of the areola. Note also the congenital cleft in the nipple.

experienced 27 abscesses and had 15 operations before the correct diagnosis was made.

Pathogenesis

Normal breast ducts are composed of 2 cell layers of cuboidal epithelium. In patients with ZD, the terminal ducts within the nipple almost always contain multiple layers of squamous metaplasia. Keratin, which is secreted by the squamous epithelial cells, fills and plugs the lumen of the ducts (**Fig. 3**). The pathological findings are strikingly similar to those of ruptured epidermal inclusion cysts, and some reports of ruptured subareolar inclusion cysts in the literature are likely ZD that has been misinterpreted by the pathologist.[23–25] There are 2 conditions that are known to be associated with squamous metaplasia of the nipple ducts with keratin plugging—smoking and congenitally cleft nipples.

Smoking

The association between cigarette smoking and ZD was first reported by Schäfer, and colleagues,[16] in 1988. They found that 90% of patients with the disease smoked or had a history of heavy smoking compared with 37% of matched controls. Others have confirmed the association with smoking.[17,19] Zhang and colleagues,[26] reported that only 2.6% of patients smoked, but over half of their patients had excision of a mass without a history of abscess or fistula, and no histologic evidence was given that indicated they had findings typically seen in the syndrome. Thirty-seven percent of their patients had nipple retraction.

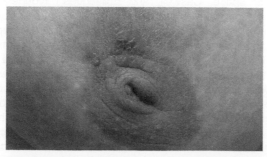

Fig. 2. Fistula at border of areola. Note fistulous opening at 11:30 position. Note congenital cleft in the central portion of nipple.

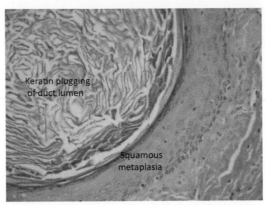

Fig. 3. Terminal duct in nipple. The normal two cell layers of cuboidal epithelium in the duct wall have been replaced with multiple layers of squamous epithelium. Keratin secretions fill the duct lumen.

Some authors have proposed that smoking leads to toxins in breast fluid that directly damage breast ducts,[17] and metabolites of nicotine have been documented to be in breast fluid after smoking.[27] Meguid, and colleagues,[18] found that 23 of their 24 patients (96%) smoked, and they postulated that vitamin A deficiency might be etiologic in the development of squamous metaplasia. It has been known for a long time that the deprivation of Vitamin A in laboratory animals results in the replacement of normal epithelium with stratified keratinizing epithelium.[28–30] There is evidence that levels of beta-carotene (a vitamin A precursor) and other plasma carotenoids are lower in people who smoke than in those who do not.[31–33] Subsequent laboratory experiments,[34] however, have demonstrated that pharmacologic doses of beta-carotene actually increase keratinized squamous metaplasia, so the role of beta-carotene deficiency, if any, in the development of squamous metaplasia remains unclear.

Congenital cleft nipple

Many patients with ZD have had a congenital cleft in the central portion of their nipples for as long as they can remember (see **Figs. 1** and **2**). Atkins first made the association between congenital nipple inversion and ZD in 1955, noting that it was present in 19 of 28 (68%) of his reported cases.[5] He postulated that the nipple inversion made it difficult for secretions to drain, causing them to build up in the duct and become infected, eventually building enough pressure to drain through the nipple orifice or rupture into the surrounding subareolar space. Caswell, and colleagues,[6] independently noted the association between congenital nipple inversion and ZD in 1956 and attributed the development of infection to "maceration" that occurred in the depth of the nipple groove. Persistent moisture in the depths of the nipple crevice with subsequent low-grade inflammation seems likely as a source of squamous metaplasia in adjacent ducts as it is known that chronic irritation can lead to squamous metaplasia.[35] Caswell reported 6 patients who had multiple unsuccessful procedures for ZD before the causative role of fistulous tracts connecting with the surface in the groove of the cleft nipples was realized.[6] Excision of the fistulous tract with the correction of the inverted nipple was successful in all 6 patients. Others have also noted the presence of nipple inversion.[17] Although nipple retraction can occur from multiple inflammatory events and scarring from previous operations, many reports of nipple retraction attributed to such causes in the literature are likely unrecognized congenital deformities.

Nipple piercing

There have been increasing reports in the literature over the last few decades that nipple piercing leads to delayed development of subareolar abscesses,[36] some of which are caused by organisms not usually seen in the breast. There have been 2 reports of patients infected with mycobacteria[37,38] and one with gonococcus.[39] David, and colleagues,[40] found that patients with nipple rings required more aspirations for abscess resolution than those without nipple rings. There has been one report of recurrence following an operation that was required because of nipple piercing,[36] but Gollapalli, and colleagues,[19] did not find a relationship between nipple piercing and an increased risk of recurrence following the treatment of the initial abscess.

The pathogenesis of abscess formation following nipple piercing seems to be a disruption of nipple ducts which allows entry of bacteria along with scarring of the ducts. There have been no reports to date as to whether squamous metaplasia and keratin plugging occur in patients with nipple piercing. It is unclear at this time whether these patients will experience recurrent problems and, if so, whether successful treatment can be accomplished by the removal of the device or will require excision of the central ducts within the nipple.

Nonoperative treatment

Cessation of smoking

The surgeon should discuss the association of smoking with the disease process with those patients who smoke. There are many health-related reasons for patients to stop smoking, and that should be encouraged. There are no good data, though, to suggest that the cessation of smoking will alter the course of the disease once the squamous metaplasia and keratin plugging have been established and symptoms have developed. It is likely it would decrease the likelihood of problems developing in other ducts or in the contralateral breast. As always, the surgeon should take care not to be judgmental, shaming the patient for "causing" the problem and adding guilt to her already exasperating symptoms. There is no reason to delay an operation in hopes that the patient will stop smoking. Most of the time she will probably not be able to stop, and in the author's experience, smoking does not seem to interfere with healing in these patients.

Antibiotics

Antibiotics play an important role in the management of ZD, whether the patient is seen at the first onset of disease or after recurrent disease when operative intervention is necessary. Several authors[11,18,41] have reported that the organism associated with first-time subareolar abscesses was *Staphylococcus*, but mixed flora and anaerobes were associated with recurrences. Multiple authors have found associations between anaerobic organisms and subareolar abscesses,[42] nipple retraction,[43] and smoking.[17–19,44,45] Russell, and colleagues,[46] found that the combination of clindamycin and flucloxacillin gave excellent coverage for all categories of breast infections. Moazzez, and colleagues,[47] found that the best oral broad-spectrum coverage for breast abscesses was provided by trimethoprim-sulfamethoxazole, but anaerobic coverage such as metronidazole should be added while awaiting culture results from recurrent abscesses, particularly if needle aspiration is conducted and the abscess cavity is left intact to heal without being exposed to oxygen.

Aspiration of abscess

If antibiotics do not prevent the development of an abscess or if one is present at the patient's initial presentation, the next step depends on the nature of the abscess. If the cavity is not extremely superficial, and relatively normal skin overlies it, aspiration frequently allows resolution and has been shown in a randomized trial to allow more rapid healing than open drainage.[48] Although there is a tendency to go straight to incision and drainage with abscesses greater than 3 cm in diameter, there is evidence that aspiration can be successful even in larger abscesses.[40] Although aspiration can be conducted with palpation alone, the use of ultrasound facilitates complete emptying and irrigation of the cavity in addition to monitoring for reaccumulation of pus.[49,50] It is sometimes necessary to aspirate the cavity several times over a 7–10 day period to achieve resolution.

A typical sonographic appearance of a subareolar abscess is shown in **Fig. 4**. Before aspiration, local anesthetic should be generously infiltrated around the abscess cavity. A three-way stopcock and intravenous tubing can be used, but a simple, cost-effective method is to introduce a 16 or 18-gauge needle on a syringe into the cavity (**Fig. 5**A) and aspirate the pus. Once the pus is evacuated, the needle can be grasped with a hemostat, and the pus-filled syringe can be replaced with one filled with lidocaine (**Fig. 5**B). Even though local anesthetic has been widely injected, the patient will still experience pain if the cavity is vigorously distended with saline. The lidocaine should be slowly instilled into the cavity to allow pain-free distention. After a moment, the cavity can then be thoroughly irrigated by swishing the lidocaine into and out of the cavity (**Fig. 5**C).

Incision and drainage

If the patient presents with a superficial abscess that has thin, attenuated skin overlying it, it is best to proceed with a simple incision and drainage in the office under local anesthesia. There is usually no need to make a large incision, insert a drain, or pack the wound. Evacuation of the pus that is pointing at the skin allows antibiotics to resolve the remainder of the phlegmon.

Operative management

Lannin[10] reported that antibiotics, aspiration, or incision and drainage resolved the problem in 33 of 67 patients (49%), so it is best not to proceed to definitive surgery if the patient has no history of previous treatment failures and does not have an established fistula. If the patient gives a history of recent treatment of the problem, has a fistula, or recurs within a few months of initial treatment, it is probably best to proceed with a definitive operation once the acute inflammation has resolved, especially if there is a congenital cleft in the nipple.

There are no randomized trials or even large series in the literature to give definitive guidance on the technical aspects of a curative operation, but there is now general

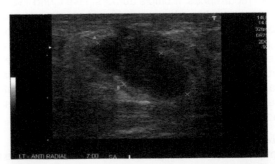

Fig. 4. Sonographic appearance of subareolar abscess. Note the fairly well-circumscribed, heterogenous, hypoechoic mass.

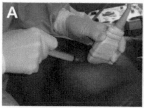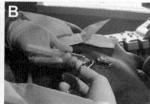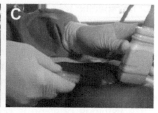

Fig. 5. Ultrasound-guided aspiration of abscess. (*A*) Large bore needle is inserted into abscess cavity and the pus is aspirated. (*B*) Needle held in place with hemostat while pus-filled syringe is replaced with one filled with lidocaine. (*C*) After slowly distending cavity, the lidocaine is vigorously swished in and out to thoroughly irrigate the abscess cavity.

agreement that the *sine qua non* for the resolution of the problem is to remove the keratin plugged ducts in and immediately below the central core of the nipple.[3,10,11,18] A cleft or inverted nipple should also be corrected at the time of duct excision.[6,12] The unresolved issue is whether this goal is best accomplished through a circumareolar incision utilized by Dixon[51] or a radial elliptical incision advocated by Lannin.[10]

Dixon reported that 91% of circumareolar wounds healed primarily, and Lannin had a 62% success rate with primary healing when using a circumareolar incision (**Table 1**). When Lannin switched from a circumareolar to a radial elliptical approach, he found that 100% of 26 wounds healed without complication.[10] Recurrence required ipsilateral re-excision in 25% of Lannin's circumareolar experience but in only 8% when a radial elliptical excision was used (Donald Lannin, MD, e-mail communication, October, 2021). Dixon reported ipsilateral re-excision in 1 of 43 patients (2%) using a circumareolar incision.

After the publication of Lannin's series in 2004, the author adopted radial elliptical excision as the routine surgical approach for these patients. The primary reason for that choice is the ability to better obliterate the dead space and allow primary healing of a closed surgical wound. Three years after adopting that approach, results were reviewed in preparation for a talk at the annual meeting of the American Society of Breast Surgeons (see **Table 1**). Eighteen patients had radial elliptical incisions, and all healed primarily without wound complications. One patient (6%) recurred in another area of the ipsilateral areola and healed primarily after a second radial elliptical excision (unpublished data). The author's results over the next decade mirrored those obtained during the three-year period, but records are not available for review.

Radial elliptical excision
Radial elliptical excision is an outpatient procedure and is best conducted during a quiescent period when there is no active infection or inflammation. There are no

Table 1				
Healing and recurrence rates for primary wound closure according to incision type				
Author/ Year	Procedures	Incision	Primary Healing	Ipsilateral Recurrence/ Re-Excision
Dixon 1991	43	Circumareolar	39/43 (91%)	1/43 (2%)
Lannin 2004	8	Circumareolar	5/8 (62%)	2/8 (25%)
Lannin 2004	26	Radial elliptical	26/26 (100%)	2/26 (8%)
Snider 2008	18	Radial elliptical	18/18 (100%)	1/18 (6%)

studies specific to ZD to guide perioperative antibiotic usage. Because of the possibility of viable bacteria persisting in the tissue or fistulous tract, these operations should not be considered to be clean. The author started trimethoprim-sulfamethoxazole and metronidazole 24 hours before the operation and continued both for 7 days afterward. With 100% primary wound healing, it was difficult to rationalize the modification of the regimen to see if equal success could be achieved with a shorter course of antibiotics.

If a fistulous opening is present at the border of the areola, a lacrimal probe is passed from the opening out through the central portion of the nipple or vice versa (**Fig. 6**). Note the white keratin alongside the probe in the image. A surgical marker is used to outline an ellipse beginning just beyond the fistulous opening and extending up onto the central part of the nipple. If no fistula is present, one can usually feel an indurated area where the pathology is located and can draw a similar ellipse around the area of induration and up onto the nipple.

If a lacrimal probe is successfully inserted, it serves as a good "handle" to elevate the tissue and give traction for dissection. An incision is made in the elliptical markings with a scalpel, then electrocautery is used beneath the skin. The process is superficial, and there is no need to dissect deeply into the breast tissue. It is usually easy to distinguish chronically scarred tissue from normal tissue, and the dissection should be at that junction without any effort to get a wide margin around the scarred or inflamed tissue.

ZD is a multi-duct process, and any attempt to limit the dissection in the nipple to a single duct is ill-advised and invites recurrence in a separate quadrant. Most, if not all, of the ducts in the central core of the nipple, can be removed along with some overlying "skin," leaving a rim of the peripheral part of the nipple to be reconstructed.

Once the specimen (**Fig. 7**) is removed, the author's preference is to irrigate the wound with dilute povidone-iodine solution to reduce the chance that viable bacteria survive in the wound, a technique also recommended by Zhang.[26] Irrigation with saline then removes the povidone-iodine before closure. The wound is closed completely without drains or wicks, taking care to obliterate the dead space with absorbable sutures. Particular attention needs to be paid to nipple reconstruction whether a cleft had been present or not. A suture should be placed at the base of the nipple

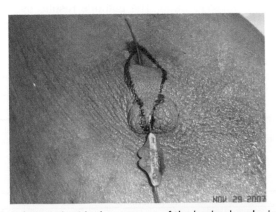

Fig. 6. Note the white keratin beside the entrance of the lacrimal probe into the nipple. The probe is useful as a retractor to put the tissue planes under tension for dissection. During nipple reconstruction, it is important to approximate points A and B at the base of the nipple to ensure nipple elevation and symmetry.

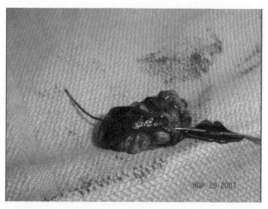

Fig. 7. The specimen is removed en bloc with the probe passing through the fistula (if present). The superficial nature of the process does not require the removal of a large amount of tissue.

reapproximating the cut edges where the ellipse came onto the nipple (see points A and B in **Fig. 6**). This suture is helpful in ensuring nipple protrusion and symmetry. The remainder of the nipple should then be closed in a manner that ensures that it protrudes. Nonabsorbable interrupted sutures that go deep enough to obliterate nipple dead space work well but require removal. A separate purse string suture might be necessary immediately beneath the nipple in some cases to prevent inversion. Within a few weeks, the nipple will have a relatively normal appearance despite the removal of the central ducts (**Fig. 8**).

If a nipple cleft is present, the inverted portion of the nipple should be excised, again leaving ample peripheral nipple for reconstruction. The excision is easy to accomplish if the indurated area or fistulous tract extends in a plane along the longitudinal axis of the crevice (**Fig. 9**). The elliptical markings encompass the inverted portion of the nipple. If the indurated area or fistula is at right angles to the crevice, the ellipse can stop at the base of the nipple and extend linearly up the side of the nipple to give exposure to the inverted portion which is to be removed (**Fig. 10**).

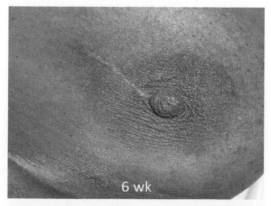

Fig. 8. The linear scar extends from the breast beyond the previous fistulous opening up onto the anterior surface of the reconstructed nipple. Note the symmetry and protrusion of the nipple. Over time the scar fades and becomes less noticeable.

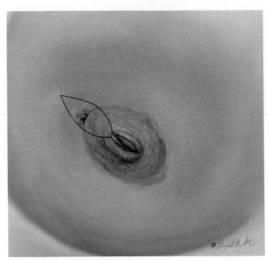

Fig. 9. Incision lines for radial elliptical excision Note the extension of the incision line along the edges of the nipple cleft which is parallel to the plane of excision.

Future Directions

It has recently been proposed that the etiology of ZD might be a chronic inflammatory process of the pilosebaceous follicles in the periareolar region similar to hidradenitis suppurativa, rather than distal obstruction from keratin plugging, and an alternative treatment was studied.[52] Eighteen fistulas were treated with ultrasound-guided percutaneous needle electrolysis which produces a nonthermal electrochemical reaction that releases caustic sodium hydroxide molecules that lead to localized tissue ablation. The authors reported success in 88% of patients, although multiple treatments were frequently required, and the follow-up was relatively short. The high degree of

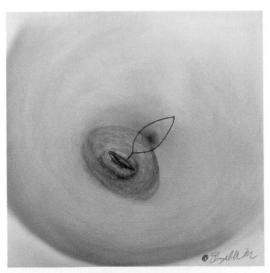

Fig. 10. Incision lines for radial elliptical excision Note the incision must be modified if the nipple crevice is perpendicular to the plane of excision.

success in procedures that remove the terminal ducts and the high failure rate for procedures that do not remove the terminal ducts or correct a cleft nipple argue against the long-term success of the new procedure. More studies are needed before it can be considered a treatment option at this time.

PERIPHERAL NONLACTATIONAL ABSCESS

Peripheral nonlactational breast abscesses are similar to soft tissue abscesses that occur elsewhere in the body. The incidence is increased by obesity and diabetes, and the most common organism is *Staphylococcus aureus*. Resistant forms are becoming increasingly more common. These abscesses generally respond to antibiotics and aspiration or drainage, and the risk of recurrence is generally low. Lam, and colleagues,[53] extensively reviewed the literature concerning the proper management of breast abscesses and concluded that needle aspiration with or without ultrasound guidance should be the first method of treatment in addition to antibiotics. Their recommendation was based on the avoidance of general anesthesia, superior cosmetic results, and a shorter healing time compared with incision and drainage. Multiple aspirations over a period of days were often necessary, and larger abscesses sometimes required percutaneous catheter placement.

SUMMARY

Peripheral nonlactational abscesses behave like other soft tissue abscesses and resolve with drainage and antibiotics. Recurrence is uncommon. Subareolar abscesses tend to recur or to develop fistulae between obstructed ducts and the border of the areola and are usually seen in women in their thirties who have a history of smoking or a congenitally cleft nipple. The underlying cause of subareolar abscesses and fistulae is the obstruction of terminal ducts due to keratin plugging secondary to squamous metaplasia of the ducts. Successful resolution of the problem requires excision of the terminal ducts in, and just below, the nipple along with the correction of nipple deformity, if present.

CLINICS CARE POINTS

- Peripheral nonlactational abscesses respond well to antibiotics and drainage with a low risk of recurrence.
- Failure to excise the keratin-obstructed terminal lactiferous ducts will lead to a high risk of recurrence of subareolar abscesses and fistulae.
- The offending ducts can be removed with a circumareolar incision or with a radial elliptical excision, closing the wound primarily without wicks or drains.
- There is no need to require the patient to stop smoking before proceeding with a definitive operation during a quiescent period.

ACKNOWLEDGMENTS

Medical illustrations were provided by Elizabeth McGowin, emcgowin3@gmail.com, (334) 322-4450.

REFERENCES

1. Ekland D, Zeigler M. Abscess in the nonlactating breast. Arch Surg 1973;107: 398–401.

2. Zuska J, Crile G, Ayres W. Fistulas of lactiferous ducts. Am J Surg 1951;81:312–9.
3. Passaro M, Broughan T, Sebek B, et al. Lactiferous fistula. Am Coll Surg 1994; 178:29–32.
4. Kilgore A, Fleming R. Abscesses of the breast: recurring lesions in the areolar area. Calif Med 1952;77(3):190–1.
5. Atkins H. Mammillary fistula. Br Med J 1955;2:1473–4.
6. Caswell H, Burnett W. Chronic recurrent breast abscess secondary to inversion of the nipple. Surg Gynecol Obstet 1956;102:439–42.
7. Crile G, Chatty E. Squamous metaplasia of lactiferous ducts. Arch Surg 1971; 102:533–4.
8. Dixon J. Periductal mastitis/duct ectasia. World J Surg 1989;13:715–20.
9. Dixon J, Ravisekar O, Chetty U, et al. Periductal mastitis and duct ectasia: different conditions with different aetiologies. Br J Surg 1996;83:820–2.
10. Lannin D. Twenty-two year experience with recurring subareolar abscess and lactiferous duct fistula treated by a single breast surgeon. Am J Surg 2004; 188:407–10.
11. Versluijs-Ossewaarde F, Roumen R, Goris R. Subareolar breast abscesses: characteristics and results of surgical treatment. Breast J 2005;11(3):179–82.
12. Li S, Grant C, Degnim A, et al. Surgical management of recurrent subareolar breast abscesses: Mayo Clinic experience. Am J Surg 2006;192:528–9.
13. Johnson S, Kaoutzanis C, Schaub G. Male Zuska's disease. BMJ Case Rep 2014; 2014. https://doi.org/10.1136/bcr-2013-201922. bcr2013201922.
14. Kazama T, Tabei I, Sekine C, et al. Subareolar breast abscess in male patients: a report of two patients with a literature review. Surg Case Rep 2017;3:128. https://doi.org/10.1186/s40792-017-0402-3.
15. Alqahtani S. A subareolar breast abscess in a man: a case report and literature review. J Taibah Univ Med Sci 2020;15(6):557–60.
16. Schäfer P, Fürrer C, Mermillod B. An association of cigarette smoking with recurrent subareolar breast abscess. Int J Epidemiol 1988;17:810–3.
17. Bundred N, Dover M, Corley S, et al. Breast abscesses and cigarette smoking. Br J Surg 1992;79:58–9.
18. Meguid M, Oler A, Numann P, et al. Pathogenesis-based treatment of recurring subareolar breast abscesses. Surgery 1995;118:775–82.
19. Gollapalli V, Liao J, Dudakovic A, et al. Risk factors for development and recurrence of primary breast abscesses. J Am Coll Surg 2010;211(1):41–8.
20. Powell B, Maull K, Sachatello C. Recurrent subareolar abscess of the breast and squamous metaplasia of the lactiferous ducts: a clinical syndrome. South Med J 1977;70(8):935–7.
21. Hanavadi S, Pereira G, Mansel R. How mammillary fistulas should be managed. Breast J 2005;11(4):254–6.
22. Lambert M, Betts C, Sellwood R. Mamillary fistula. Br J Surg 1986;73:367–8.
23. Suk J, Woo G. Clinical and Imaging Features of a ruptured epidermal inclusion cyst in the subareolar area: a case report. Am J Case Rep 2019;20:580–6.
24. Naftali Y, Shoufani A, Krausz J, et al. Unusual presentation of epidermoid cyst mimicking breast cancer involving the areola—case report. Int J Surg Case Rep 2018;51:17–20.
25. Singh M, Maheshwari B, Khurana N, et al. Epidermal inclusion cyst in breast: Is it so rare? J Cytol 2012;29(3):169–72.
26. Zhang Y, Zhou Y, Mao F, et al. Clinical characteristics, classification and surgical treatment of periductal mastitis. J Thorac Dis 2018;10(4):2420–7.

27. Hill P, Wynder E. Nicotine and cotinine in breast fluid. Cancer Lett 1979;6(4–5): 251–4.
28. Wolbach S, Howe P. Tissue changes following deprivation of fat-soluble A vitamin. J Exp Med 1925;42:753–77.
29. Malloy C, Laskin J. Effect of retinoid deficiency on keratin expression in mouse bladder. Exp Mol Pathol 1988;49(1):128–40.
30. Liang F-X, Bosland M, Huang H, et al. Cellular basis of urothelial squamous meta-plasia. J Cell Biol 2005;171(5):835–44.
31. Menkes M, Comstock G, Vuilleumien J, et al. Serum beta-carotene, vitamins A and E, selenium and risk of cancer. N Engl J Med 1986;315:1250–4.
32. Chow C, Thacker A, Changchit C, et al. Lower levels of vitamin C and carotenes in plasma of cigarette smokers. J Am Coll Nutr 1986;5:305–12.
33. Russel-Briefel R, Bates M, Kuller L. The relationship of plasma carotenoids to health and biochemical factors in middle-aged men. Am J Epidemiol 1985; 122(5):741–9.
34. Liu C, Wang X, Bronson R, et al. Effects of physiological versus pharmacological beta-carotene supplementation on cell proliferation and histopathological changes in the lungs of cigarette smoke-exposed ferrets. Carcinogenesis 2000;12:2245–53.
35. Alonso F, Campos R, Sanz I, et al. Conservative management of unusual kerati-nising squamous metaplasia of the bladder in a 28-year-old female and overview of the literature. Case Rep Urol 2012. https://doi.org/10.1155/2012/940269. Article ID 940269. 3 pages.
36. Jacobs V, Golombeck K, Jonat W, Kiechle M. Mastitis nonpuerperalis after nipple piercing: time to act. Int J Fertil Womens Med 2003;48(5):226–31.
37. Siddique N, Roy M, Ahmad S. Mycobacterium fortuitum abscess following breast nipple piercing. ID Cases 2020;28:21.
38. Pearlman M. Mycobacterium chelonei breast abscess associated the nipple piercing. Infect Dis Obstet Gynecol 1995;3(3):116–8.
39. Ceniceros A, Galen B, Madaline T. Gonococcal breast abscess. ID Cases 2019; 9:18.
40. David M, Handa P, Castaldi M. Predictors of outcomes in managing breast ab-scesses—a large retrospective single-center analysis. Breast J 2018;24:755–63.
41. Oliveira V, Cubas-Vega N, Del-Teio P, et al. Non-lactational infectious mastitis in the Americas: a systematic review. Front Med (Lausanne) 2021;8:672513. https://doi.org/10.3389/fmed.2021.672513.
42. Leach R, Eykyn S, Phillips I, et al. Anaerobic subareolar breast abscess. Lancet 1979;1(8106):35–7.
43. Leach R, Eykyn S, Phillips I. Vaginal manipulation and anaerobic breast ab-scesses. Br Med J (Clin Res Ed) 1981;282(6264):610–1.
44. Bharat A, Gao F, Aft R, et al. Predictors of primary breast abscesses and recur-rence. World J Surg 2009;33(12):2582–6.
45. Bartolome-Alvarez J, Solves-Ferriz V. Microbiology of breast abscesses. Enferm Infecc Microbiol Clin (Engl Ed) 2021. https://doi.org/10.1016/j.eimc.2021.01.004. S0213-005X(21)00024-0.
46. Russell S, Neary C, Elwahab S, et al. Breast infections—microbiology and treat-ment in an era of antibiotic resistance. Surgeon 2020;18(1):1–7.
47. Moazzez A, Kelso R, Towfigh S, et al. Breast abscess bacteriologic features in the era of community-acquired methicillin-resistant *Staphylococcus aureus* epi-demics. Arch Surg 2007;142(9):881–4.

48. Naeem M, Rahimnaijad M, Rahimnaijad N, et al. Comparison of incision and drainage against needle aspiration for the treatment of breast abscess. Am Surg 2012;78(11):1224–7.
49. Fahrni M, Schwarz E, Stadlmann S, et al. Breast abscesses: diagnosis, treatment and outcome. Breast Care (Basel) 2012;7(1):32–8.
50. Dhamija E, Singh R, Mishra S, et al. Image-guided breast interventions: biopsy and beyond. Indian J Radiol Imaging 2021;31(2):391–9.
51. Dixon J, Thompson A. Effective surgical treatment for mammary duct fistula. Br J Surg 1991;78(10):1185–6.
52. Berna-Serna J, Garcia-Vidal J, Escolar-Reina M. A new treatment for mamillary fistulas using ultrasound-guided percutaneous needle electrolysis. J Clin Med 2020;9(3):649.
53. Lam E, Chan T, Wiseman S. Breast abscess: evidence based management recommendations. Expert Rev Anti Infect.Ther 2014;12(7):753–62.

Moving?

Make sure your subscription moves with you!

To notify us of your new address, find your **Clinics Account Number** (located on your mailing label above your name), and contact customer service at:

Email: **journalscustomerservice-usa@elsevier.com**

800-654-2452 (subscribers in the U.S. & Canada)
314-447-8871 (subscribers outside of the U.S. & Canada)

Fax number: **314-447-8029**

**Elsevier Health Sciences Division
Subscription Customer Service
3251 Riverport Lane
Maryland Heights, MO 63043**

*To ensure uninterrupted delivery of your subscription, please notify us at least 4 weeks in advance of move.

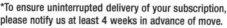

Printed and bound by CPI Group (UK) Ltd, Croydon, CR0 4YY

03/10/2024

01040471-0019